TAI CHI
illustrated

Master Pixiang Qiu

Weimo Zhu

Human Kinetics

Library of Congress Cataloging-in-Publication Data

Qiu, Pixiang.
 Tai chi illustrated / Master Pixiang Qiu and Weimo Zhu.
  p. cm.
 Includes bibliographical references.
1. Tai chi. I. Zhu, Weimo, 1955- II. Title.
 GV504.Q58 2012
 613.7'148--dc23

                      2012025530

ISBN-10: 1-4504-0160-0 (print)
ISBN-13: 978-1-4504-0160-9 (print)

The web addresses cited in this text were current as of August 2012, unless otherwise noted.

Acquisitions Editor: Tom Heine; **Developmental Editor:** Laura Floch; **Assistant Editor:** Elizabeth Evans; **Copyeditor:** Alisha Jeddeloh; **Permissions Manager:** Martha Gullo; **Graphic Designer:** Nancy Rasmus; **Graphic Artist:** Kim McFarland; **Cover Designer:** Keith Blomberg; **Photographs (cover and interior):** Neil Bernstein; **Visual Production Assistant:** Joyce Brumfield; **Photo Production Manager:** Jason Allen; **Art Manager:** Kelly Hendren; **Associate Art Manager:** Alan L. Wilborn; **Illustrations:** © Human Kinetics; **Printer:** Versa Press

Printed in the United States of America   10 9 8 7 6 5 4 3 2 1

The paper in this book is certified under a sustainable forestry program.

Human Kinetics
Website: www.HumanKinetics.com

United States: Human Kinetics
P.O. Box 5076
Champaign, IL 61825-5076
800-747-4457
e-mail: humank@hkusa.com

Canada: Human Kinetics
475 Devonshire Road Unit 100
Windsor, ON N8Y 2L5
800-465-7301 (in Canada only)
e-mail: info@hkcanada.com

Europe: Human Kinetics
107 Bradford Road
Stanningley
Leeds LS28 6AT, United Kingdom
+44 (0) 113 255 5665
e-mail: hk@hkeurope.com

Australia: Human Kinetics
57A Price Avenue
Lower Mitcham, South Australia 5062
08 8372 0999
e-mail: info@hkaustralia.com

New Zealand: Human Kinetics
P.O. Box 80
Torrens Park, South Australia 5062
0800 222 062
e-mail: info@hknewzealand.com

E5291

To our wives, Guilin Xu and Enyi Cai,
and our families for their love and support always

Contents

Preface

Tai chi, a Chinese mind–body exercise, was developed as a form of martial arts in China around the 12th century AD. It is an exercise based on the Chinese Tao philosophy of yin–yang balance, the only such exercise in the world. In fact, all its movements and applications reflect Tao philosophy. Over time, people began to use tai chi mainly for health purposes; now millions of people worldwide practice it regularly. Tai chi practitioners move their bodies in a slow, relaxed, and graceful manner through a series. Tai chi has been proven to have beneficial effects with respect to balance, fall prevention, and nonvertebral fractures, as well as many chronic diseases. In the 1990s, the Western research community started to examine the effectiveness of tai chi interventions using scientific research methods and standardized outcome measures. Tai chi is quickly becoming one of the most popular mind–body exercises in the West.

In *Tai Chi Illustrated*, key stances, foot patterns, and single forms are depicted with the use of more than 15 color illustrations so that beginners can learn tai chi easily. By combining forms, two routines (one with six forms and another with twelve forms) are presented and illustrated. Finally, basics and key movements of push hands, in which two people practice tai chi movements in a manner similar to its origins in martial arts, are introduced and illustrated.

Tai Chi Illustrated is organized into five parts. Part I includes five chapters. Chapter 1 provides a comprehensive introduction to tai chi, including its history, unique movement features, relationships with the philosophy of Chinese Tao and Chinese medicine, various styles and schools of tai chi, and known health benefits. Chapter 2 covers basic posture, chapter 3 presents basic foot movements, chapter 4 covers basic hand forms and movement, and chapter 5 describes basic stances. Part II consists of four chapters. Chapter 6 introduces three forms for cardiovascular health, chapter 7 introduces three forms for stress relief and low-back health, chapter 8 introduces two forms for balance, and chapter 9 introduces two forms for coordination. Part III consists of the three remaining chapters. Chapter 10 introduces a six-form routine, chapter 11 introduces a twelve-form routine, and chapter 12 presents several push hands routines.

The primary audience for this book is anyone interested in mind–body exercises, such as tai chi and yoga. It is especially aimed at beginning to intermediate tai chi practitioners but should also be useful to people interested in exploring holistic health activities, including physical educators, personal trainers, and physical therapists, along with those seeking alternative and complementary treatments for chronic health conditions such as heart disease and depression.

Read the book, learn tai chi, improve your health, and enjoy life!

Acknowledgments

No book can be put together without the support of many, and this is especially true for *Tai Chi Illustrated*. We want to acknowledge and thank Heidi Krahling and Dong (Steve) Zhu for their many hours of careful and skillful proofreading. We thank models Dong (Steve) Zhu, Elena Boiarskaia, and Sara Khosravi Nasr for their hard work. Thank you to Leta Alverri Burch for her input on early chapter drafts and to Wei Wang and Wei-Guo Ma for their assistance during the initial development of the book draft. We also want to thank the Human Kinetics staff for their assistance in developing and producing this book, especially Tom Heine and Jason Muzinic for their initial support and guidance in development, Laura Floch for her diligent work as the development editor, Neil Bernstein for his excellent photos, and Doug Fink for his videography. We extend our gratitude to the Shanghai University of Sports, especially the Wu Shu and Humanities Colleges and the University of Illinois at Urbana-Champaign for their support. Finally, we both thank our families for their unwavering love and support.

part I

Tai Chi Basics

Chapter 1, which provides a comprehensive introduction to tai chi, includes the history of tai chi, its unique features, and its relationship with Chinese Tao philosophy and traditional Chinese medicine. Various styles and schools of tai chi, as well as known health benefits, are also introduced. Chapters 2 to 5 detail basic tai chi movements. Chapter 2 introduces basic postures of tai chi, chapter 3 teaches basic foot movements, chapter 4 covers basic hand forms and movements, and chapter 5 introduces basic stances of tai chi.

chapter 1

Art and Practice of Tai Chi

Tai chi, or more correctly tai chi quan (or tai ji quan using the Chinese spelling system), is a Chinese mind–body exercise that is rapidly becoming popular in the United States. Derived from Chinese martial arts and Tao philosophy, tai chi is a unique Chinese mind–body exercise that has centuries of history. Some practitioners refer to it as *moving meditation. Mind–body exercise* is typically defined as a physical exercise executed with a profoundly inward focus. Although there is an assortment of mind–body exercises, tai chi is the only one that itself is a philosophy. More important, it is a recognized part of Chinese medicine and has been proven to provide many health benefits. It requires no equipment and little space, and it can be practiced anytime, anywhere, and by anyone, including older adults and people with chronic diseases.

Because of its rich cultural history, philosophical foundation, and accessibility to almost everyone, tai chi is becoming one of the most popular forms of exercise not only in China but around the world.

People in more than 150 countries practice tai chi. It is estimated that more than 2.5 billion people practice tai chi regularly, making it the most popular Chinese mind–body exercise. In some countries, such as Japan, tai chi is already as popular as it is in China, and many practitioners in those countries have reached high skill levels.

Tai chi has become an important vehicle for introducing and promoting Chinese culture around the world. In 2006, Tai chi was selected to be part of the first group in China's national intangible cultural heritage (ICH), a system for protecting cultural identities and therefore the cultural diversity of humankind. The Chinese government applied to the United Nations Educational, Scientific and Cultural Organization (UNESCO) for tai chi to be part of UNESCO's ICH in 2009.

What Is Tai Chi Quan?

Tai chi quan (pronounced "tai-chi-chwon") is a form of Chinese boxing based on tai chi philosophy. *Quan* means "fist" in Chinese. In martial arts, it refers to various forms of boxing, and each form has its own offensive and defensive fighting style that involves varying dynamic and static elements, from moving back and forth to a combination of firm and soft moves. Quan can be considered a martial art performed without equipment, or more simply Chinese boxing. Because the movement in tai chi quan is similar to a moving river—long, relaxed, and continuous—tai chi quan is also known as a long, soft, continuous form of Chinese boxing.

Before beginning tai chi quan, one stands still and the body enters into a state of *wuji* (e.g., body weight is balanced between both legs). As soon as the practice starts, the body enters into tai chi, that is, a constant exchange of yin and yang, with body weight being constantly moved from the firm (yang) leg to the empty (yin) leg. The tai chi principle is also applied to fighting using tai chi quan. When an opponent's hit (yang) is coming, a tai chi master never directly fights back because yang to yang is not balanced and he would likely get hurt even if he were stronger than his opponent. Rather, a tai chi master always tries to use his opponent's own strength to cause the opponent to lose balance.

It is believed that the Chen style, the oldest style of tai chi quan, was created by Master Chen (Chen, Wangting), a retired general at the end of the Ming Dynasty (1368-1644). He spent his retirement living a tranquil life in the country. During the farming season, he was busy working on his farm, but he practiced boxing during the off-season. His boxing practice was initially for health purposes in order to regulate the yin–yang of the body and help the circulation of Qi and blood. (*Qi* or *chi* refers to vital energy in Chinese medicine and will be explained in more detail later in this chapter.) Meanwhile, he was also teaching his children and grandchildren how to use boxing as exercise and how to keep a balanced diet. Through his exercise and diet practice, he believed that one could live a peaceful, healthy, and harmonious life. The development of tai chi, that is, the modification of a martial art from use on the battlefield to an exercise for well-being, reflected the general's desire to return to nature and to live a life that reflected harmony between man and nature.

The Chen style of tai chi quan is full of tai chi principles (i.e., yin–yang contrasts and interconnections). For example, the mind should be at peace while the body is actively moving during tai chi practice, there is a constant change between firmness and looseness in the continual transfer of weight from one leg to the other and the opening and closing of the arms while coordinating movements with inhaling and exhaling, and the end of a movement flows smoothly into the beginning of another movement. Recognizing the movements' unique connection with tai chi philosophy, Master Wang (Wang, Zongyue), a well-known martial arts master at the beginning of the Qing Dynasty (1644-1912) who also was well versed in philosophy, studied tai chi and provided an excellent summary of tai chi quan in his book *Tai Chi Quan Theory* *(*translated also as the *Tai Chi Treatise)*, which remains popular today. From then on, *tai chi quan* or simply *tai chi* became the official name of this exercise form. Because many movements in tai chi are based on tai chi philosophy, many people believe that practicing tai chi regularly will help them achieve balance or harmony with nature.

Characteristics of Tai Chi Movements

Tai chi is an exercise with four distinct movement characteristics:

1. *Movements are soft and continuous.* Movements mimic a slow-moving river.

2. *Movements are calm and quiet.* While doing tai chi, you pursue a sense or being of calmness. Again, similar to a slow-moving river, often you do not feel the movement but rather the calmness. This sensation is especially true in your mind. The Chinese believe that if you relax your mind, your qi will become calm and quiet. Even while moving, every piece of the movement is felt as if you were static—the movement begins smoothly and slowly progresses through a succession of thousands of static poses.

3. *Movements are relaxed.* The principle of being relaxed applies to all movements. To relax, you must relax the whole body and move in a natural way. Do not use any extraneous strength or energy. Again, you must have a relaxed mind to have a relaxed body. Mental peace is important because it is often associated with your outlook and attitude toward life.

4. *Movements are circular.* The movements in tai chi are rarely straightforward or angular, and this is especially true for the arm movements. Instead, tai chi movements follow paths of circles or curves. Tai chi masters often say that all tai chi movements can be summarized by circles, which fits perfectly within the general concept of tai chi philosophy, as we'll learn later in this book—the movements create patterns of repeated circles.

Tai Chi and Traditional Chinese Medicine Theories

Traditional Chinese medicine (TCM) is well known for many of its practices, such as herbs and acupuncture, and many of its theories, including yin–yang, five elements, qi or vital energy, and blood, meridians, and internal organs as a system. The foundation of TCM is aligned with tai chi theory. People are considered as a whole and their balance (yin and yang) are key elements in TCM diagnosis and treatment. In addition, TCM believes that heath is directly related to one's qi level (the higher, the better) and circulation along the meridian system (the more qi movement, the better). Although there are still many unanswered questions concerning the meridian system, it has been proven to have a relationship with health. Fostering qi, promoting qi and blood circulation, and dredging the meridians have always been the focus of TCM treatments.

Tai chi breathing routines and many of its movements are associated with TCM. For example, transferring weight from one leg to another during tai chi practice is directly related to the change from yang to yin and vice versa. In line with "Exercise is medicine," a slogan of the American College of Sports Medicine (ACSM), one may say that "Tai chi is Chinese medicine."

Yin and Yang

Tai chi (see figure 1.1 for the Chinese characters) is a concept in Chinese philosophy that has had a great influence on Chinese culture. Its name abounds with meaning. It is believed that the earliest appearance of tai chi was in the *I Ching*, or *Book of Changes*, a well-known Chinese philosophy book written in the third century BC. The tai chi characters in Chinese represent the Tao philosophy, or Taoism, which believes that, although the world is full of contrasts or conflicts, it can reach harmony by balancing those contrasts or conflicts.

According to the Tao, the contrasts or conflicts in nature can be best summarized using the yin and yang concepts. The direct meanings of yin and yang in Chinese are the bright side and the dark side of an object. Note that the concepts of *bright* and *dark* do not have the Western cultural connotation of *good* and *bad* in Tao philosophy. The Tao philosophy uses yin and yang to represent a wide range of opposite properties in the universe: cold and hot, slow and fast, still and moving, masculine and feminine, lower and upper, and so on. In general, the characteristics of stillness, descent, darkness, erosion, slowness, and

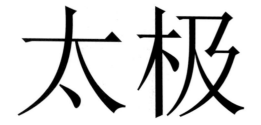

Figure 1.1 Chinese characters for *tai chi.*

organic diseases pertain to yin, and in contrast, movement, ascent, brightness, growth, energy, and functional diseases pertain to yang. Yin and yang are opposites yet complementary; they do not exist independently of each other but rather are able to change, or morph, into each other. For example, day (yang) turns into night (yin) and winter (yin) turns into spring (yang). The internal forces or rules of nature lead to the harmony of yin and yang and are the Tao, or way. In the *Book of Changes*, tai chi or Tao is the integration of yin and yang, the contrary forces interconnected and interdependent in nature.

> According to medical science, diseases can be classified into two general groups: organic and functional. Organic diseases are those in which an actual destruction of bodily tissue has occurred (e.g., blood diseases, cancer, tuberculosis), whereas functional diseases are caused by temporary disturbances of function and there is no actual loss or structural alteration of tissue (e.g., arthritis, balance disorder, dementia).

In TCM, health is represented as a balance of yin and yang, although the balance of yin and yang in a healthy body is not always perfect. Under normal circumstances, the yin and yang balance in the body is in a state of constant change based on both the external and internal environment. For example, while exercising, a person's body is more energized and has greater yang, and once exercising stops and a quiet, peaceful state is entered, yin dominates. Illness is caused by an imbalance of yin and yang in the body. The treatment of illness in TCM therefore is the process of rebalancing yin and yang in the body. This is done through the use of acupuncture, herbal remedies, exercise, diet, and lifestyle changes (e.g., smoking cessation). As balance is restored in the body, so is health restored. Balance in TCM includes balance in both physical and mental health.

The character *tai* in Chinese derives from the character *dai*, meaning "big." To represent something that is much larger than just being big, the ancient Chinese added a stroke inside the *dai* character to create the *tai* character. Thus, *tai* refers to the largest or most supreme (see figure 1.2 for a comparison of the characters). The character *chi*, as shown in figure 1.3, originally referred to the highest section, or peak, of a roof. Placing both of these Chinese characters together into *tai chi* (see figure 1.1) synergizes their meanings into a new meaning that refers to the universe or something that is immense.

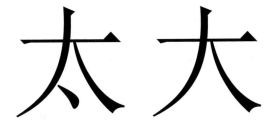

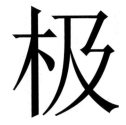

Figure 1.2   Chinese characters for *tai* and *dai*.

Figure 1.3   Chinese character for *chi*.

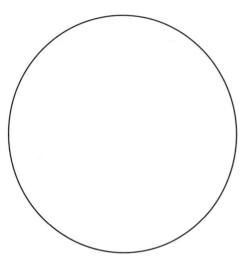

Figure 1.4 Wuji diagram.

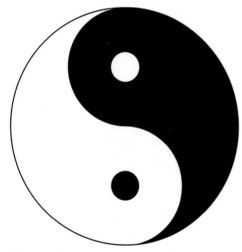

Figure 1.5 Yin and yang diagram.

It is believed that Tuan Chen (872-989 AD), a Taoist during the end of the Five Dynasties and Ten Kingdoms period (907-960 AD) and at the beginning of the Northern Song Dynasty (960-1127 AD), created the earliest wuji diagram, which is simply a circle (see figure 1.4). The circle represents the original status of the universe in which everything was static. Later, Dunyi Zhou (1017-1073 AD), a philosopher during the Northern Song Dynasty, published a short, well-known article called "Tai Chi Diagram," in which the tai chi concept was further described and extended. Basically, the ancient Chinese believed that the universe was originally a static entity without yin or yang. Later, the yang element came into existence through some mysterious and dynamic movement of qi, or vital energy. The end or extreme of the yang dynamic movement is stillness, which produced yin. Life and the world were then created as a result of the movement and exchange of yin and yang.

Wuji does not include the yin and yang concept, yet tai chi can be considered a special form of wuji, one that includes the balancing of yin and yang. Zhou's descriptions of tai chi can be better represented by the yin and yang diagram (see figure 1.5). In the diagram, yin and yang are symbolized by a circle consisting of two semicircular teardrops, a white one representing yang (sun, male, fire, and so on) and a black one representing yin (moon, female, water, and so on). The black spot inside the white teardrop and the white spot inside the black teardrop symbolize that yin and yang are not absolutes; they change or morph into each other (e.g., the end of day begins night). In its entirety, this symbol of yin and yang also represents the balance and change of tai chi within the universe, nature, and even society. Tai chi therefore reflects the mechanism of the universe.

Qi and the Meridians

Qi (pronounced "chi") in Chinese medicine is considered to be vital energy, or life force. Although its existence has not been completely confirmed by modern science, it is generally believed that qi circulates along the body's meridians, whose existence has been confirmed by modern biophysics (Chen, 2004). A meridian, according to TCM, is a path through which the life energy known as qi is believed to flow. There are 20 meridians in the body, including 12 regular channels or meridians and 8 extraordinary channels or meridians. The 12 regular meridians each correspond to an internal organ, nourishing the organ and extending to an extremity (see figure 1.6). There are 649 acupuncture points on the meridians. Meridians are also divided into yin and yang groups. For example, the yin meridians of the arm are Lung, Heart, and Pericardium meridians, and the yang meridians of the arm are the Large Intestine, Small Intestine, and Triple Heater.

The smooth circulation of qi within the meridians helps maintain health. Qi and the meridians can benefit from tai chi practice because tai chi emphasizes relaxation of the mind during practice, which in turn aids the circulation of qi. In addition, it is believed that the relaxed manner of tai chi movements improves the ability of the meridians to nourish organs and tissues. Finally, tai chi movement, such as waist rotation and limb flexion and extension, could function as a kind of self-massage, which should stimulate qi and strengthen the physiological function of tissues and organs.

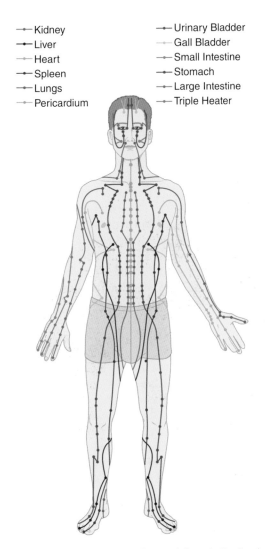

- Kidney
- Liver
- Heart
- Spleen
- Lungs
- Pericardium
- Urinary Bladder
- Gall Bladder
- Small Intestine
- Stomach
- Large Intestine
- Triple Heater

Figure 1.6 Twelve regular meridians in the body.

Although there is still a long way to go to understand how meridians work, more and more scientific evidence is being accumulated to support its existence and role in maintaining health. As an example, there is growing interest in acupuncture, which is based on the meridians. It is believed that medical effectiveness, cost effectiveness, and credibility provided by clinical trials and physiological research are the key reasons for the growing interest in acupuncture (Stux & Hammerschlag, 2001).

Five Elements Theory

The back-and-forth footwork of tai chi is believed to connect with the Five Elements theory, which posits wood, fire, earth, metal, and water as the basic elements of the material world. The theory of Five Elements is an ancient philosophical concept used to explain the composition and phenomena of the physical universe. In TCM, the theory is used to interpret the relationship between the physiology and pathology of the human body and the natural environment. For example, when a person's heart, an element of fire, has a problem, the cause could originate from the kidneys, an element of water, since water restrains fire. As in yin–yang theory, the five elements are interdependent and are constantly moving and changing (see figure 1.7).

The ancient Chinese philosopher Laozi declared, "Nature is the law," thousands of years ago, and this remains a key concept in Eastern culture. As mentioned earlier, tai chi is the martial art whose development was influenced the most by traditional Chinese philosophy. There is a saying about this particular aspect of tai chi: "Every part of the human body is tai chi; the contrast and harmony of the dynamic and static movements of the body is a reflection of tai chi." One should relax while practicing tai chi by breathing naturally and performing movements according to the feedback one's body provides. When practicing tai chi outside in nature (e.g., beside a lake, in a forest, on grass) and in the fresh air, there is likely a feeling that nature is the law and a focus on the connection between one's mind and soul with nature; thus, it is easy to relieve stress and enjoy the relaxation and flow between body and mind. In return, one should achieve better health and a peaceful mind. In fact, tai chi theory and practice open up a new way of thinking that promotes practitioners' balance with nature so that they may live a more harmonious and ecological life.

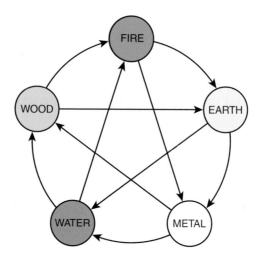

Figure 1.7 Five Elements relationship diagram.

Tai Chi Styles and Schools

China is a huge country, and travel during ancient times was inconvenient. As a result, each region formed its own distinct culture. Because of limited interaction among people of various regions, family heritages, legacies, and traditions feature strongly in the long history of Chinese culture. In all of these areas, regions, and families, many styles and schools of various professions and skills were formed. The great variety of Chinese cuisines is a perfect example of the cultural diversity across China. The same is also true for tai chi styles or schools. Named after families, the most popular tai chi styles are Chen, Yang, Wu (Z-Q), Sun, and Wu (Y-H) (Although the spelling of *Wu* is the same, they are two different Chinese characters, so to distinguish between them in English, the initials of their first names were added.) These styles are briefly described next.

Chen

The Chen style is the oldest type of tai chi. Created by the retired general Chen (Chen, Wangting; 1600-1680), Chen style is known for its combination of both soft and firm, as well as quick and slow, movements. Occasionally, explosive strength and a strong foot and leg pushing are used. It is a style that maintains many boxing features used in fighting on battlefields.

Yang

Created by Master Yang (Yang, Luchan; 1799-1872), Yang style is known for its standardized format, slow and relaxed movements, and soft and continuous style. Because it is easy to learn and the movements are beautiful to observe, it is the most popular style of tai chi, and it is the one taught in this book.

Wu (Z-Q)

Wu (Z-Q) style is modified from the Yang style and features a small range of quick yet relaxed movements. The upper body is slightly inclined forward during practice. The key master who developed this style was Master Wu (Wu, Zhen-Quan; 1870-1942).

Sun

Sun style was developed by combining the skills and methods of other Chinese martial arts, specifically Xingyiquan and Baguazhang, into tai chi. As a result, its footwork moves much faster and it contains more frequent back-and-forth movements. In addition, its transitions are often combined with open–close movements (i.e., transferring body weight from one leg to the other while the arms are open). The key master who developed this style was Master Sun (Sun, Lutang; 1860-1933).

Wu (Y-H)

The Wu (Y-H) style is known for its slow and relatively small range of movements, lesser bending of the knee, and limited reach of hands and arms. The person responsible for this Wu style was Master Wu (Wu, Yu-Hsiang; 1812-1880).

Later, to meet the needs of the general public, many more variations of tai chi were developed. For example, to help the general public learn tai chi, the Chinese government developed and promoted a 24-form simplified tai chi in the 1950s; later, routines with 48 and 88 forms of tai chi, based mainly on the Yang style, were offered. Because of the rich history of tai chi, many tai chi styles, including several subvarieties within styles, and forms are practiced both in China and around the world. Special forms of tai chi have also been developed specifically for a population or an aesthetic purpose, such as in the case of wheelchair tai chi and tai chi fan, which involves holding a fan during tai chi practice. There even are tai chi routines that exist purely for the purpose of competition.

Tai Chi and Health

The industrial and information revolutions changed the world. Although they brought many advances to civilization, they also brought many social problems, including competition and its related stress and increased isolation among people. Their negative effects on health and well-being are significant and well documented. Fortunately, tai chi can be used to buffer these negative effects. For example, tai chi can help young people achieve relaxation and bring their bodies and minds into balance, and for older adults who practice together, as many do every morning in China, tai chi serves as a social network, a place and time to make new friends and provide social support.

Tai chi is part of TCM, and its significant impact on health has been well documented. Although tai chi was introduced to the United States in the 1970s, an interest in its health benefits did not start until Dr. Steven L. Wolf and his team published their balance study in 1996 (Wolf, Barnhart, Kutner, McNeely, Coogler, & Xu, 1996). Their subjects were 162 women and 38 men with an average age of 76.2 who were free of debilitating conditions such as crippling arthritis, Parkinson's disease, and stroke. The researchers divided the subjects into three groups: One group performed a simplified 10-form version of tai chi, one group received biofeedback-based training in balance on a movable platform, and one group received education about falls but no physical training. The tai chi and biofeedback groups were given 15 weeks of training, and researchers kept track of the participants' reported falls for four months.

After the intervention, the tai chi subjects reduced their falling risk by an average of 47.5 percent compared with the other groups. Since the publication of that study, interest in tai chi and its health benefits has continued to grow. Hundreds of studies have now been published and interest has extended to many other health areas, such as the impact of tai chi on physical function, quality of life, and cardiovascular diseases. In addition, many tai chi books have been published, including some with a research focus (e.g., Hong, 2008).

According to a recent review (Zhu et al., 2010) of 25 reviews, which included hundreds of studies from around the world, tai chi has been demonstrated to be a useful exercise for a variety of chronic diseases and conditions, including Parkinson's disease, osteoarthritis, rheumatoid arthritis, high blood pressure, cancer, cardiovascular disease, diabetes, a propensity toward falling, and so on. In addition, tai chi practice has been shown to be beneficial to overall health, balance and control, bone mineral density, psychological and mental status, and aerobic capacity. A few highlights are summarized here.

Overall Health

Tai chi has the potential to improve many of the physiological and psychological aspects of chronic conditions, and it is also a safe and effective intervention for promoting balance, cardiorespiratory fitness, and flexibility in older adults. Tai chi has been shown to be effective as an aerobic exercise in reducing blood pressure, reducing the risk of falls, and increasing function in older adults.

Balance and Control

Moderate evidence supports using tai chi to improve balance and postural stability, indicating that it is a reasonable intervention for clinical use. It has also been found that tai chi improves balance in older adults, although it was not shown to be effective at reducing the rate of falls in older populations. Studies have shown that health outcomes associated with postural control could benefit from tai chi practice.

Although not all studies supported tai chi in fall prevention for older adults, a number of studies found tai chi to be effective in reducing the fear of falling, meaning that interventions aimed at improving older adults' self-efficacy regarding falls could use tai chi. Meanwhile, tai chi was found to be useful for preventing falls in relatively young, prefrail older adults. In addition, although more rigorous studies are needed to make any assertions about the use of tai chi for Parkinson's patients, there is favorable evidence in support of using tai chi to help people with Parkinson's disease.

Osteoarthritis

There is promising evidence in support of using tai chi to reduce pain associated with osteoarthritis, and there are even larger effect sizes in pain reduction from tai chi compared with other popular interventions, such as nonsteroidal anti-inflammatory drugs (NSAIDs). Also, the review found that tai chi may be beneficial for improving the balance and physical function of people with osteoarthritis.

Rheumatoid Arthritis

Tai chi improved ankle plantar flexion in people with rheumatoid arthritis, but most other measures, such as activities of daily living and swollen joints, showed no improvements after tai chi interventions. None of the studies indicated any harmful effects of tai chi practice, and the review reported that adherence rates in the tai chi interventions were higher than in the controls, indicating that subjects may enjoy participating in tai chi over other exercises. Some studies also found that tai chi interventions could improve the pain, fatigue, mood, depression, vitality, and disability index of people with rheumatoid arthritis.

Bone Mineral Density

Tai chi has been found to be a promising intervention for maintaining bone mineral density in postmenopausal women. No significant adverse effects of practicing tai chi were reported, and research also indicates that tai chi may improve other risk factors associated with low bone mineral density. Additionally, it was found that tai chi interventions did increase bone mineral density in postmenopausal women compared with a no-treatment control group.

Psychological Health

Tai chi has been found to increase well-being and self-efficacy as well as improve overall mood. Tai chi was also a safer choice of exercise for those who were deconditioned or had exercise intolerance.

Blood Pressure

Many studies have reported that a tai chi intervention could lead to lower blood pressure. In all the studies, tai chi was shown to be safe and had no adverse effects.

Cancer

Tai chi has been useful as a complement to traditional cancer treatment. Tai chi helped improve the self-esteem and health-related quality of life, function in activities of daily life, and shoulder range of motion of cancer survivors. In addition, tai chi has been shown to increase the immune response as well as psychological function of cancer survivors.

Cardiovascular Disease

Most studies for this population reported improvement with tai chi interventions, such as lower blood pressure and greater exercise capacity. In addition, no adverse effects were reported. These studies concluded that tai chi may be a beneficial adjunctive therapy for patients with cardiovascular disease.

Aerobic Capacity

Tai chi is an effective exercise to improve aerobic capacity. Statistically significant and large effect sizes ($ES = 1.33$) were noted in the cross-section studies, meaning that subjects experienced significant aerobic improvements from practicing tai chi. On the other hand, small effect sizes were found within the experimental studies ($ES = 0.38$). Studies comparing sedentary people with tai chi participants also noted larger effects when tai chi was practiced for at least a year. It has been concluded that tai chi could be used as an alternative form of aerobic exercise, and further inquiry is recommended in this area.

Practice Tips for Learning Tai Chi

Compared with most exercises, tai chi requires no equipment and little space, and it can be done at anytime. The following tips may be helpful for tai chi beginners.

Am I ready?

If you are planning to start an exercise program or become much more physically active than you are now, it is a good idea for you to answer the following seven questions from the Physical Activity Readiness Questionnaire (PAR-Q):

1. Has your doctor ever said that you have a heart condition and that you should only do physical activity recommended by a doctor?

2. Do you feel pain in your chest when you do physical activity?

3. In the past month, have you had chest pain when you were not doing physical activity?

4. Do you lose your balance because of dizziness or do you ever lose consciousness?

5. Do you have a bone or joint problem (for example, back, knee, or hip) that could be made worse by a change in your physical activity?

6. Is your doctor currently prescribing drugs (for example, water pills) for your blood pressure or heart condition?

7. Do you know any of other reason why you should not do physical activity?

If you answered "Yes" to any of these questions, you should talk with your doctor before starting a physical activity program or becoming much more physically active.

Source: Physical Activity Readiness Questionnaire (PAR-Q) © 2002. Used with permission from the Canadian Society for Exercise Physiology www.csep.ca.

What do I wear to practice tai chi?

There are no specific requirements other than wearing clothing that is loose and comfortable. There are also no specific requirements for shoes; any exercise shoes or comfortable shoes with low heels are fine.

When should I practice tai chi?

The best time of the day to practice is in the morning for easier adherence since there is less chance of interruption of practice time first thing in the morning. Other times are also fine, but you should wait at least 30 minutes after eating a heavy meal.

How often and for how long should I practice tai chi?

To get the best results, 30 to 60 minutes is the best length for practice, but any time is better than no time. Just 5 to 10 minutes of practice (especially the stances) here and there will also be beneficial. Ideally, you should practice every day. Try to practice tai chi at least three times a week.

(continued)

(continued)

Where should I practice tai chi?

Outside in nature in the fresh air is best, but practice anywhere you can, such as in your office when taking a break.

Can I combine tai chi with other exercises?

Tai chi can integrate with other exercises easily. If you already have a regular exercise routine, you can link it with your tai chi practice. For example, you can practice tai chi as part of your cool-down after running.

In this chapter, you learned what tai chi is, including its historical roots, relationship with Chinese Tao philosophy and traditional Chinese medicine theories, its movement characteristics, and different styles and schools. More important, you learned the health benefits of practicing tai chi. This book, through a step-by-step approach and illustrations, is designed to help you learn tai chi in an easy and enjoyable way. In chapter 2, you will learn some basic postures; then some basic foot movements in chapter 3; basic hand forms and movements in chapter 4, and basic stances in chapter 5. Then, in chapters 6-9, you will learn some of the most popular tai chi forms: forms for cardiovascular health (chapter 6), forms for stress management and lower back health (chapter 7), forms for balance (chapter 8), and forms for coordination (chapter 9). In chapters 10 and 11, you will learn routines with the above forms connected together. You will learn a simple 6-form routine in chapter 10 and a slightly more difficult 12-form routine in chapter 11. Finally, in chapter 12, you will learn push hands, practicing tai chi with another person.

Learn and enjoy tai chi!

chapter 2

Basic Posture

Remembering how the hands, elbows, arms, feet, legs, and torso move simultaneously is one of the major challenges when starting tai chi. Rather than rushing into learning tai chi forms and routines and getting confused and frustrated, you will start by learning some basic tai chi movements. In this chapter, you will learn how to maintain correct postures and move the upper body correctly. In chapter 3, you will then move on to the basic tai chi movements of the legs and feet, and finally, you will start learning the basic movements of the arms and hands in chapter 4.

Tai chi differs from many Western exercises in that its movements are performed in a natural and relaxed manner. To learn tai chi quickly and accurately, an understanding of the principles of tai chi postures is essential. This chapter introduces the major components of tai chi postures from head to knee. After describing and illustrating the key elements of each posture and its related principles, common mistakes in these postures are described and illustrated. Errors are a part of learning, and recognizing them early and not allowing them to become habit is important when learning new motor skills, particularly when learning on your own. We therefore have provided some common mistakes and how to correct them. It is a good idea to practice in front of a mirror when learning tai chi so that you can have visual feedback.

Additionally, through hundreds of years of teaching, learning, and practice, Chinese tai chi masters have summarized key technical essentials of major tai chi postures and movements into tai chi sayings. We will present these corresponding sayings in Tai Chi Saying sections throughout the chapters. Make sure you pay attention to the key points mentioned in these sayings.

Head

During tai chi practice, the head should remain straight and upright with the neck straight, and the head should not incline in any direction. This position should be held in a natural, straight manner rather than in an exaggerated, extended position. The eyes look naturally forward in tai chi positions and head movement is coordinated with hand movements. See figure 2.1a for an illustration of head position from a front view and figure 2.1b for this position from a side view.

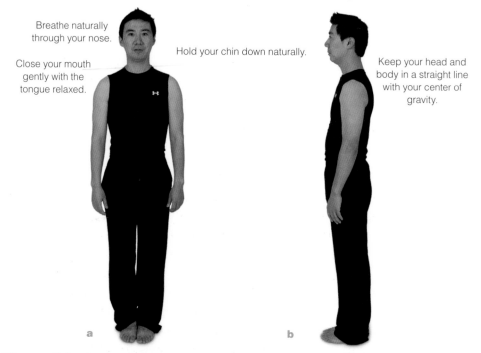

Breathe naturally through your nose.

Close your mouth gently with the tongue relaxed.

Hold your chin down naturally.

Keep your head and body in a straight line with your center of gravity.

a

b

Figure 2.1   Correct head position: (a) front view and (b) side view.

Common mistakes of the head position are inclining the head to the front or back too much (see figure 2.2, a and b) and tilting it to the left or right (see figure 2.2c). To correct the head when it is inclined back too far, return the head to an upright position with the chin held down. In contrast, if the head is inclined forward too much, return the head to an upright position by lifting the chin. If the head is tilted to the left or right, correct it by returning the head to the center. One easy way to avoid mistakes with the head position is to experience various head positions in front of a mirror and try to remember how it feels when the head is in the upright position. Getting feedback from other practitioners may also be helpful.

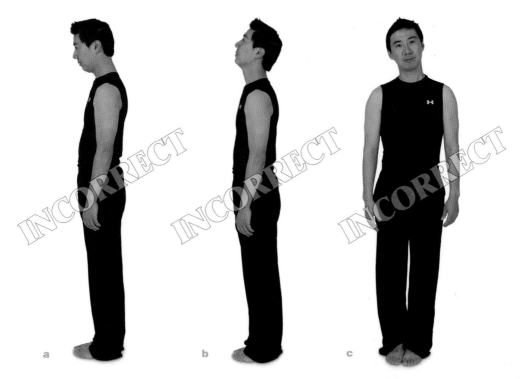

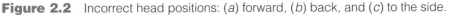

Figure 2.2 Incorrect head positions: (*a*) forward, (*b*) back, and (*c*) to the side.

Tai Chi Saying: *Xu Ling Ding Jing*

Meaning: Most Chinese sayings consist of four characters. In this saying, *xu* means "empty" or "lightly," *ling* means "to lead," *ding* means "top," and *jing* means "strength." Together, this saying means to imagine a string is holding your head up. In other words, you should have the feeling that there is a string coming from the top of your head that is slightly pulling so as to keep your head up and straight. This is one of the fundamental technical aspects of tai chi practice: The head is to be held upright, but not on a stiff neck. In addition, head movement is to be coordinated with the movements of other parts of the body.

Shoulders and Elbows

Shoulders should remain even with each other and should be naturally down or relaxed (see figure 2.3*a*). Relaxed shoulder joints and muscles are the key to keeping the shoulders in a low, naturally relaxed position. The elbows should also be held in a low, natural, and relaxed manner (see figure 2.3*b*). There should be a distance of about one to one and half fists between your elbow and your body so that your elbows can move comfortably (recall that tai chi evolved from boxing, and elbows that are raised too high could expose your ribs for your opponent to attack). Relaxed shoulders are a must for relaxed elbows. Also, a relaxed mind is important because people tend to shrug or tighten their shoulders when nervous or agitated.

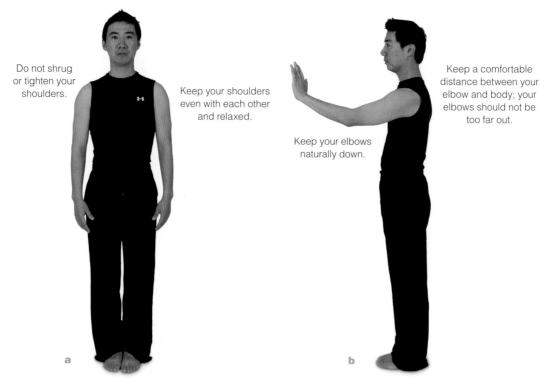

Do not shrug or tighten your shoulders.

Keep your shoulders even with each other and relaxed.

Keep your elbows naturally down.

Keep a comfortable distance between your elbow and body; your elbows should not be too far out.

a

b

Figure 2.3   Correct (*a*) shoulder and (*b*) elbow position.

Common mistakes of the shoulder position include holding the shoulders too tightly (see figure 2.4*a*) and not keeping them even (see figure 2.4*b*). When the shoulders are held too tightly, they are up close to the ears. To correct this, relax the shoulder joints and surrounding muscles. It is helpful to shrug or tighten the shoulders and then relax them several times to learn and remember how relaxed shoulders feel. When the shoulders are uneven, relax the front and back muscles of the shoulders. Practice in front of a mirror several times to make sure the shoulders are even. A common mistake with the elbow position is holding them too tightly to the body (see figure 2.5*a*) or holding them too high (see figure 2.5*b*). To correct these mistakes, relax the shoulders and elbows.

Tai Chi Saying: *Che Jian Zhui Zhou*

Meaning: *Chen* means "down," *jian* means "shoulder," *zhui* means "dropping," and *zhou* means "elbow." Together, this means to sink the shoulders and drop the elbows with a relaxed mind. Relaxed shoulders are crucial.

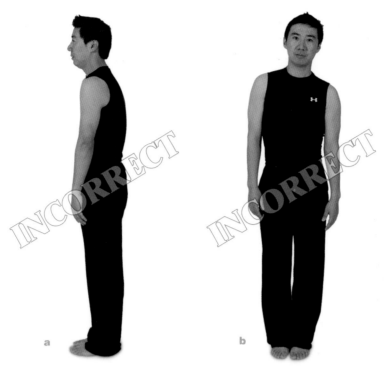

Figure 2.4 Incorrect shoulder position: (*a*) too tight and (*b*) uneven.

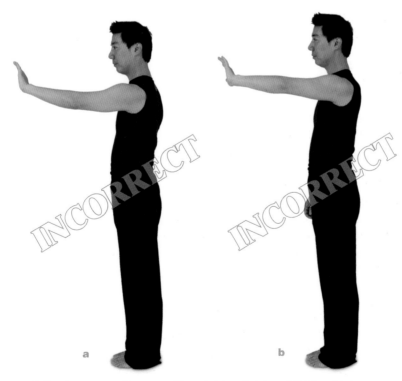

Figure 2.5 Incorrect elbow position: (*a*) too tight and (*b*) too high.

Chest and Back

During tai chi practice, you should keep your chest comfortably relaxed by holding it naturally concaved. However, this does not mean it should be sunken; rather, there should simply be a slight dip. The upper back should be relaxed, natural, and slightly convex but not hunched (see figure 2.6).

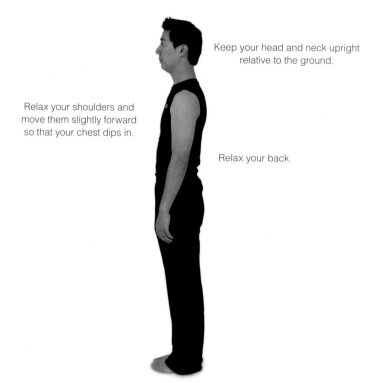

Keep your head and neck upright relative to the ground.

Relax your shoulders and move them slightly forward so that your chest dips in.

Relax your back.

Figure 2.6   Correct chest and back position.

Common mistakes concerning the upper body include holding the chest too rigidly forward (see figure 2.7a) and making it too concave so as to have a rounded back (see figure 2.7b). When the chest is too far forward and rigid, the whole body is too tight and the shoulders are not relaxed. Correct these mistakes by relaxing the upper body, including the chest, shoulders, and back, and relaxing the shoulders forward to let your chest come in a bit. When the chest is sunken in too much, the chest muscles are too relaxed. Correct this mistake by moving the shoulders back a little, tightening the chest muscles a little, and keeping the head, chest, and whole body in the same line as your center of gravity.

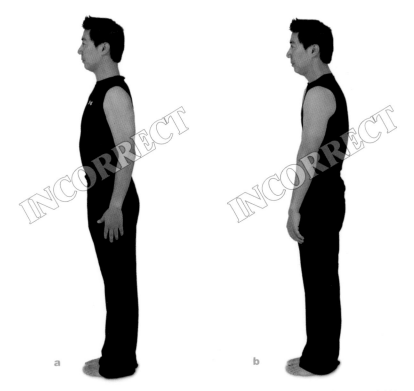

Figure 2.7 Incorrect upper-body position: (*a*) rigid, forward chest and (*b*) concave chest with a rounded back.

Tai Chi Saying: *Han Xong Ba Bei*

Meaning: *Han* means "contain" or "hold," *xong* means "chest," *ba* means "pull up," and *bei* means "back." Together, this means to arc your chest, round your back, and keep your upper body relaxed. Appropriately relaxing the chest and back is critical.

Waist and Hips

The waist should be relaxed, natural, steady, and upright (see figure 2.8). Keep the muscles around the waist relaxed and loose for movement, and do not hold your abdomen in too tightly or straight. Except for a few movements, your lumbar spine should be straight. Your hips should also be relaxed and natural yet upright in relation to the ground so that they are in line with your head and upper body (do not tuck or extend the hips). This might take some shifting from how you naturally hold them at rest.

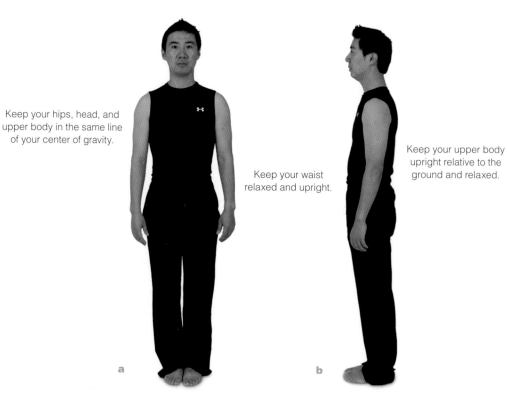

Keep your hips, head, and upper body in the same line of your center of gravity.

Keep your waist relaxed and upright.

Keep your upper body upright relative to the ground and relaxed.

Figure 2.8   Correct waist and hip position: (*a*) front and (*b*) side.

Common mistakes concerning the waist and hips include holding the waist in too tightly (see figure 2.9*a*) and extending the hips backward (see figure 2.9*b*). When the waist is held in too tightly, the chest is positioned too far forward and the back muscles are too tight. Correct these mistakes by relaxing your back and upper-body muscles and keeping your hips, upper body, and head along the same vertical line. When the hips are extended too far back, the hips, upper body, and head are not positioned along the same vertical line and the upper body tilts forward too much. Correct these mistakes by keeping the upper body upright and the hips forward along the same vertical line of your head, upper body, and waist (in the middle of your center of gravity).

Tai Chi Saying: *Shong Yao Jian Ten*

Meaning: *Shong* means "relax," *yao* means "waist," *jian* means "restrain," and *ten* means "hip." Together, this means you should have a relaxed waist and hips that are aligned with the rest of the body.

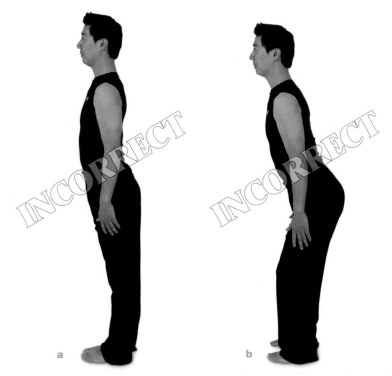

Figure 2.9 Incorrect waist and hip position: (*a*) waist held in too tight and (*b*) hips extended back.

Abdomen

The lower part of belly (see figure 2.10) is called the *Dan Tian*, and it is where the Chinese believe qi is stored. During tai chi practice, you should breathe from the abdomen, which means breathing using the diaphragm (the diaphragm moves up during exhalation and down during inhalation) instead of expanding the chest. Breathe in and out deeply and relax the abdominal area, letting it move naturally as you inhale and exhale. As a result of this type of breathing, qi will move into the Dan Tian and the lower belly should feel solid and energized. To obtain this feeling, it is necessary to maintain the previously described chest and waist positions.

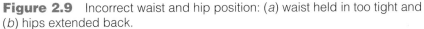

Inhale and exhale deeply with the corresponding natural breathing movements of the abdomen.

Relax your upper body.

Relax your abdomen.

Figure 2.10 Correct abdominal position.

Pelvis, Thighs, and Knees

The posture and movement of the hip, pelvis, and upper leg is important in tai chi. The Chinese call the front area of the pelvis the *dang* and the area between the thighs the *kua*. While doing tai chi movements, the hip joints and muscles should be relaxed, and the thighs should be open, ensuring a space between the thighs and knees. The knees are aligned toward the front and are bent slightly to ensure that there is a space between the thighs and knees (see figure 2.11).

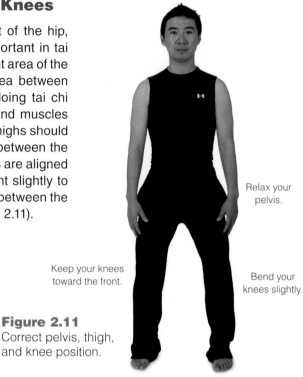

Relax your pelvis.

Bend your knees slightly.

Keep your knees toward the front.

Figure 2.11
Correct pelvis, thigh, and knee position.

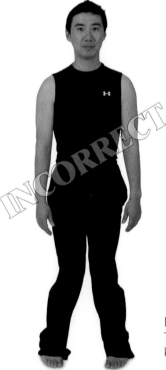

The most common mistake concerning the pelvis, thighs, and knees is not having enough space between the thighs (see figure 2.12). When there is not enough space between the thighs, the legs are too close to each other and the knees are not pointing toward the front. Correct these mistakes by standing with your legs separated, bending the knees slightly, and keeping the knees pointing forward.

Figure 2.12 Incorrect pelvis, thigh, and knee position: There is not enough space between the thighs and the knees are not forward.

Tai Chi Saying: *Yuan Dang Song Kua*

Meaning: *Yuan* means "round" or "circle," *dang* refers to the front area of the pelvis, *song* means "relax," and *kua* refers to the area between the thighs. Together, this means you should round the lower abdomen and relax the pelvis.

Short breaths (i.e., inhaling and exhaling too quickly) is a common problem. Holding your body too tightly, including both the upper body and abdomen, is another common problem. The best way to avoid these mistakes is to relax your upper body and abdomen and breathe in and out slowly and deeply. When breathing in, imagine the air in your breath going directly to the Dan Tian.

Tai Chi Saying: *Chi Chen Dantian*

Meaning: *Chi* means "vital energy," *chen* means "sink," and *Dan Tian* refers to the lower belly, where chi is believed to be stored. Together, this means to focus the mind on the lower belly (Dan Tian).

A journey of a thousand miles starts with a single step. You have taken the first and a very important first step in learning tai chi in this chapter. After learning basic postures, you are now ready to learn other basic tai chi movements. Keep going since the more tai chi you learn, the more enjoyable it will be.

chapter 3

Basic Foot Movements

As introduced in chapter 1, tai chi is the only exercise and the only martial art whose movements are, in themselves, a philosophy. The yin and yang belief that lies at the heart of the tai chi philosophy and movements is often represented by the balance of empty and firm movements. This is especially true for leg movements in tai chi. When one leg is firm, meaning it is supporting the body, the other leg should be empty, meaning it has just a small percentage of body weight on it. Pay attention to the firm–empty principle while learning tai chi and make sure you are always aware of which leg is firm and which leg is empty. Meanwhile, as you move and switch your body weight from one leg to the other, the firm–empty relationship constantly changes (i.e., when you are moving one leg from firm to empty, the other leg is moving from empty to firm). In most tai chi movements, these changes should be gradual. Tai chi leg movements can be classified as either step patterns, which are static, or footwork, which is kinetic. In tai chi forms or routines, the leg movements are a combination of both step patterns and footwork, which are described next.

Step Patterns

Major step patterns in tai chi are the bow step, empty step, and single-leg step. In this chapter, we will learn these steps one-by-one. After familiarizing yourself with these steps and arm movements, which will be learned in the next chapter, learning the basic forms in chapters 6-9 will become easier.

Bow Step

As the name implies, in this step pattern you stand as if you were an archery bow, with one leg in front and the other in back. The front knee is bent 45 degrees between the back of the thigh and calf, and the back leg is held straight at about 45 degrees from the body (see figure 3.1). The front foot is planted straight ahead and the back foot is at a 45-degree angle from the body. Keep about 60 percent of your body weight on the front leg and 40 percent on the back leg, and make sure your feet are not on the same line in order to create a stable base.

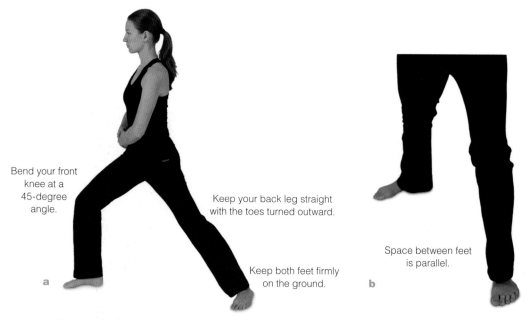

Bend your front knee at a 45-degree angle.

Keep your back leg straight with the toes turned outward.

Keep both feet firmly on the ground.

Space between feet is parallel.

a

b

Figure 3.1   Correct bow step position: (*a*) side view and (*b*) front view.

Common mistakes of the bow step include standing with the legs too close together from front to back (see figure 3.2*a*) or to the side in either direction (see figure 3.2*b*), bending the front knee too far forward over the front toes (see figure 3.2*c*), placing all weight on the front leg (see figure 3.2*d*), and pointing the back foot straight to the front with no angle (see figure 3.2*e*). Correct these mistakes by practicing with legs only first, following a straight line on the floor to make sure your legs do not cross the line, alternating legs and steps forward, and practicing bow steps with a different leg in front each time.

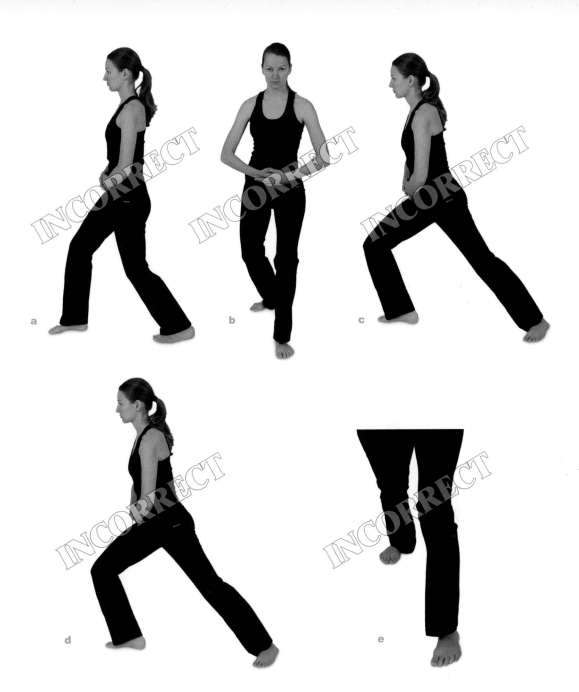

Figure 3.2 Incorrect bow step positions: (*a*) legs too close together front to back, (*b*) legs too close together laterally, (*c*) front knee bent too much, (*d*) all weight on the front leg, and (*e*) back foot pointing straight to the front.

Empty Step

Stand with one leg empty in this step pattern by moving your body weight to one leg, with the knee bent slightly and foot turned outward. Specifically, this means you stand with the back leg firm with the knee bent, carrying 90 to 95 percent of your body weight on that leg. The back foot is turned out about 45 degrees. The front leg is empty and a half step to the front, only touching the ground with the heel or toes of the foot (see figure 3.3).

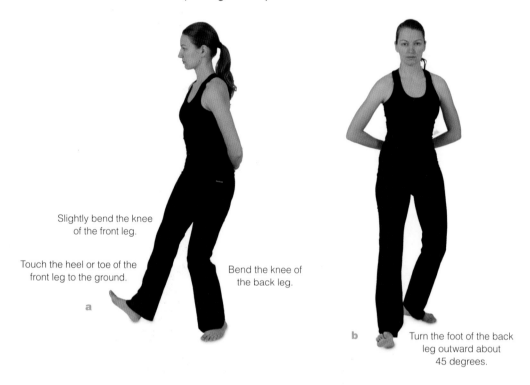

Slightly bend the knee of the front leg.

Touch the heel or toe of the front leg to the ground.

a

Bend the knee of the back leg.

b

Turn the foot of the back leg outward about 45 degrees.

Figure 3.3   Correct empty step position: (*a*) side view and (*b*) front view.

Common mistakes of the empty step include having body weight almost evenly distributed between both legs (see figure 3.4*a*), keeping the legs too close together to the front and back (see figure 3.4*b*) or to the side in either direction (see figure 3.4*c*), and placing too much of the front foot on the ground (see figure 3.4*d*). Correct the mistakes by clearly shifting the body weight onto the back leg; making sure the front foot only touches the ground with the heel or toe; practicing by standing with one leg in front and the other in back with your body weight evenly distributed between both legs; shifting your body weight slowly onto the back leg while maintaining good balance and then shifting back to sharing body weight between both legs, repeating several times to practice weight transfer; and practicing empty steps with a different leg in front each time.

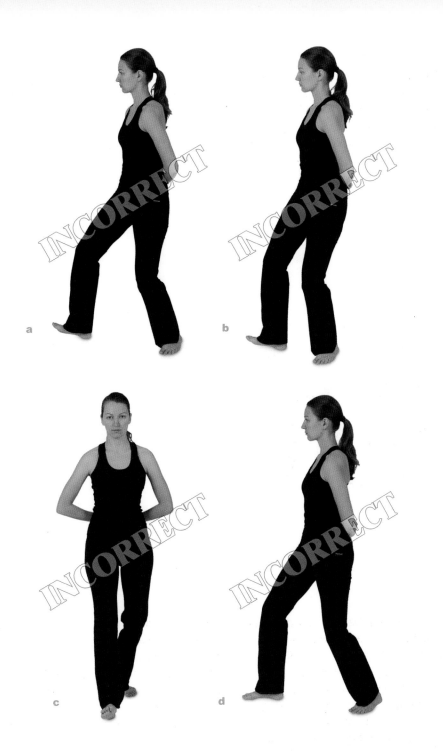

Figure 3.4 Incorrect empty step positions: (*a*) weight distributed evenly, (*b*) legs too close together front to back, (*c*) legs too close together laterally, and (*d*) too much of the front foot touching the ground.

Single-Leg Step

For this step pattern, stand on one leg, with the other leg bent and held high in front of your body (see figure 3.5). To do this, shift weight slowly onto one leg and stand wholly on this leg (you can hold onto a chair to practice in the beginning). Bend the other leg and hold it up in front of the body at about a 90-degree angle between the upper body and thigh, with the foot pointed naturally down toward the ground. The upper body should be straight and balanced.

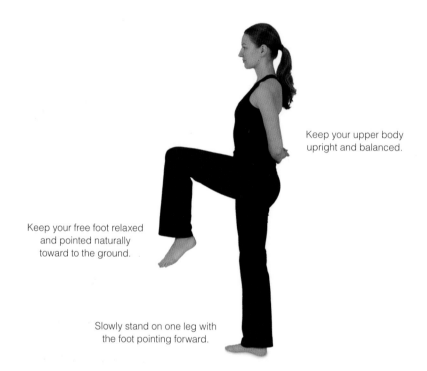

Keep your upper body upright and balanced.

Keep your free foot relaxed and pointed naturally toward to the ground.

Slowly stand on one leg with the foot pointing forward.

Figure 3.5   Correct single-leg step position.

Common mistakes of the single-leg step include raising the free leg too quickly, not pointing the standing foot toward the front but rather turning it to either side (see figure 3.6a), leaning the upper body to the front too much (see figure 3.6b), and losing your balance. Correct the mistakes by shifting your body weight to the standing leg slowly; taking the free foot off the ground slowly, just 1 or 2 inches (3-5 cm) initially from the ground to feel the balance; raising the free leg gradually when feeling in control and stable; holding for 1 to 2 minutes after the lifted thigh reaches a 90-degree angle to the upper body, with the foot pointing naturally toward the ground; returning the free leg to the ground slowly; moving the free leg up and down several more times; and switching to the initial free leg as the standing leg and repeating the previous steps several times.

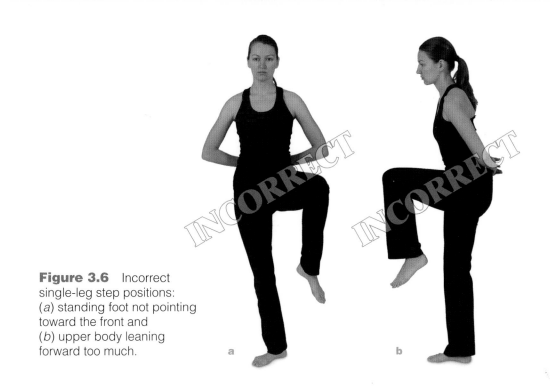

Figure 3.6 Incorrect single-leg step positions: (*a*) standing foot not pointing toward the front and (*b*) upper body leaning forward too much.

Footwork

Major footwork movements include forward, backward, side step, and follow-up. They were named based on the way the legs move.

Forward Footwork

The key principle of this movement is moving back before moving forward. You should shift your body weight from one leg to the other, moving it back and forth in a controlled manner. In this footwork, you move the non-weight-bearing leg one step to the front, touch the heel on the ground, and then set the full foot down. Shift weight gradually onto the non-weight-bearing leg.

To perform the forward footwork, start in the bow step, standing with the left leg in front and the right leg in back (see step 1); move your body weight back onto your right leg and point your left toes up (see step 2); pivot your left foot out about 30 degrees, place your foot flat on the ground, and shift your body weight gradually onto your left leg (see step 3) while moving the right leg slightly up and bringing it forward so as to place your right foot alongside the arch of the left foot, with only the toes of the right foot touching the ground (see step 4); take a half step forward with the right leg, but place only the heel of your right foot on the ground (see step 5); and shift your body weight slowly onto your right leg while your right foot lowers until it is flat on the ground (about 70 percent of your body weight is on the right leg and 30 percent on the left; see step 6). Repeat these steps several times, alternating between your left and right legs.

(continued)

Forward Footwork *(continued)*

1 Start from a left bow step with the distance of a full step between the feet; in addition, there should be about 4 inches (10 cm) horizontal distance between the left and right legs. Turn the right foot (back leg) out about 45 degrees and bend the knee of the back leg. Shift most of your body weight onto the right (back) leg and slightly bend the knee of the left (front) leg. Touch your left foot to the ground. Point your right (back) foot out at an angle of about 45 degrees.

2 Move your body weight back onto your right (back) leg and bend your right knee. Raise your left toes with your left heel still touching the ground.

3 Turn your left foot out about 30 degrees and place it flat on the ground. Shift your body weight gradually onto your left foot and leg. Bend your left knee.

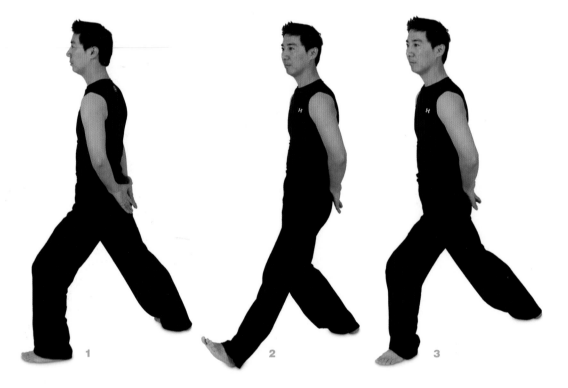

1   2   3

4 Keep your left knee bent and body weight on your left leg. Raise your right leg slightly and bring it forward. Place your right foot alongside the arch of your left foot, with the right toes touching the ground.

5 Take a half step forward with your right leg and touch your right heel to the ground. Your body weight is still on your left leg.

6 Touch the entire right foot to the ground and move most of your body weight (70 percent) slowly onto your right leg. Complete the movement by ending in a right bow step.

7 Repeat the previous steps by alternating right and left legs.

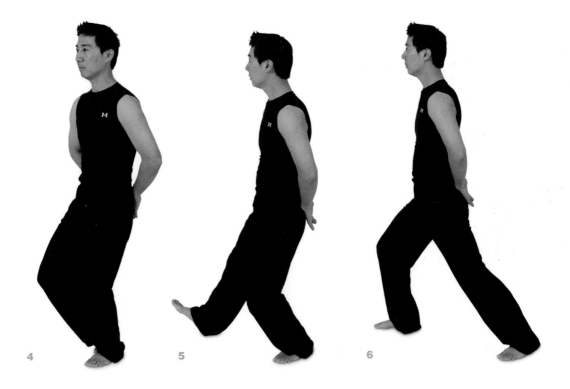

4   5   6

Common mistakes of the forward footwork include distributing body weight evenly throughout the movement, touching the ground using the whole foot instead of the heel first, and moving too quickly and not controlling for balance. Correct these mistakes by clearly transferring body weight from one leg to the other, touching the ground with your heel first, and having a stable base before transferring body weight.

Backward Footwork

This movement has several similarities with the forward footwork, including moving body weight onto one leg first, moving the non-weight-bearing leg, and then transferring weight to the non-weight-bearing leg. The key difference from the forward movement is that in the backward movement, you touch your non-weight-bearing toes (rather than your heel) on the ground first and then transfer the weight to the heel. Moving backward is a characteristic of tai chi.

To perform the backward footwork, start with your legs separated in a natural, comfortable way (see step 1); move your body weight to the right leg and then bend and lift your left leg alongside the right leg (see step 2); extend your left leg back, touching the ground with the toes first (see step 3); allow the left foot to flatten onto the ground as you move your body weight onto the left leg and move the right leg back alongside the left leg, with your right toes touching the ground (see steps 4 and 5); now, repeat steps 3 and 4 by moving the right leg back. For practice, repeat steps 2 through 5 several times and end the movement in the initial standing position from step 1.

1 Stand naturally with your legs separated and body weight divided equally between both legs.

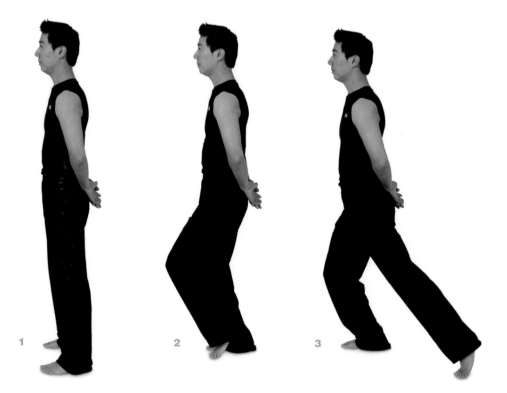

2 Shift your body weight to your right leg and raise your left heel, with your left toes touching the ground. Keep your upper body upright along the same line as the lower body.

3 Raise your left leg slightly and move it backward a half step. Touch the ground with your left toes. Keep your upper body upright.

4 Touch the entire left foot to the ground. Move your body weight simultaneously and slowly to your left leg. Move your right foot toward the arch of your left foot. Keep your upper body upright.

5 Complete the transfer of body weight to your left leg. Touch your right toes near (i.e., width of about two wrists) the arch of your left foot. Keep your upper body upright.

Common mistakes of the backward footwork include distributing body weight evenly throughout the movement, touching the ground with the whole foot instead of the toes first, and moving too quickly without having good balance control. Correct these mistakes by transferring body weight from one leg to the other, touching the ground with the toes first, and having a stable base before transferring body weight.

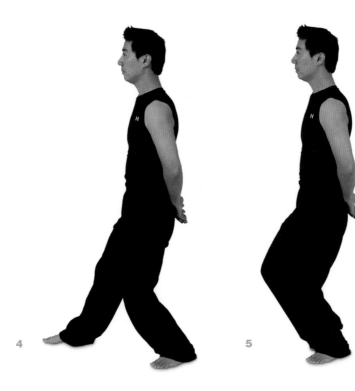

4   5

Side Step

The side step has many similarities with the backward movement, including moving the weight to one leg, touching the toes of the non-weight-bearing foot to the ground first, and transferring the weight gradually onto the non-weight-bearing leg, keeping the upper body upright during the movement. The key difference from the backward movement is that the leg movements in the side step are side to side.

To perform the side-step footwork, start with your legs separated in a natural and comfortable way (see step 1); move your body weight onto your right leg, raise the left leg slightly, take a small side step outward, and lightly touch the toes of your foot to the ground (see step 2); place your left foot fully on the ground and then slowly shift your body weight onto your left leg (see step 3); raise your right leg when your body weight has shifted entirely onto your left leg; and set your right foot down about 4 inches (10 cm) away from and parallel to your left foot (see step 4). Repeat steps 1 through 4 several times.

1 Stand naturally with your legs separated and body weight evenly distributed between both legs.

2 Move body weight onto your right leg and bend your right knee. Move your left leg a half step out to the left. Keep your upper body upright.

3 Transfer body weight to your left leg and bend your left knee. Keep your upper body upright.

4 Bring your right foot toward your left foot and stop about 4 inches (10 cm) from the left foot. Transfer body weight back onto your right leg.

Common mistakes of the side step include distributing body weight evenly throughout the movement, touching the ground using the whole foot instead of the toes first, and moving too quickly without good balance control. Correct these mistakes by clearly transferring body weight from one leg to the other, touching the ground with the toes first, and having a stable base before transferring body weight. Start with a small side step with just a slight bend in the knee of the weight-bearing leg, and gradually increase the size of the step.

Follow-Up Footwork

The name *follow-up* comes from the moving pattern of the back, trailing leg in walking. In normal walking, the back leg usually passes the front leg when taking a full step, but when performing the follow-up step, the back leg moves forward less than a half step, stopping behind the front leg.

To perform the follow-up footwork, start with your left leg in front and right leg in back, with most of your body weight on your right leg (see step 1); move your body weight forward onto your left leg (see step 2); move your right leg a half step forward (see step 3); and place your right foot slightly behind your left foot (see step 4). Return to the starting position and repeat steps 1 through 4 several times. Then, repeat the same movement several times with your right leg in front and your left leg in back.

1 Start the same as in the bow step but with more body weight on your back leg and keeping your legs separated and both feet firmly on the ground. Bend your front knee 45 degrees. Your back leg should stay straight with the foot pointing outward. Keep about 40 percent of your body weight on your front leg and 60 percent on your back leg. There should be a distance of about one fist along the line running between the feet.

2 Slowly transfer most of your body weight to your left leg and bend your left knee slightly more, but not too much. Raise your right heel, with only the toes touching the ground. Keep your upper body upright.

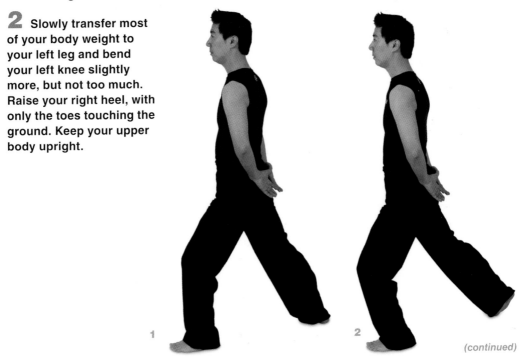

1

2

(continued)

Follow-Up Footwork *(continued)*

3 Move your body weight completely onto your left leg and move your right foot a half step forward. Lightly touch your right toes to the ground. Keep your upper body upright.

4 Put your entire right foot on the ground and transfer most of your body weight (about 70 percent) back onto right leg. Keep your upper body upright.

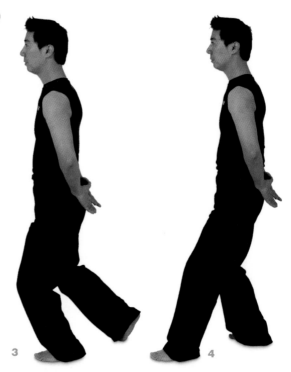

Common mistakes of the follow-up footwork include distributing your body weight almost evenly between the legs during movement; positioning the legs too close together front and back or laterally; moving without a clear transfer of weight; moving too quickly, without good balance control; and not keeping the upper body upright. Correct the mistakes by shifting your body weight from one leg to another when starting to move, transferring your body weight slowly with a stable base, and always holding upper body upright.

You have now learned some key foot movements of tai chi. One of the key principles in tai chi footwork is "Light up and light down," which means you should raise and lower your legs and feet slowly and lightly during tai chi movements. This is one of the reasons why tai chi footwork is sometimes called *cat steps*—the movement is light, soundless, controlled, stable, and fast when needed, just like a cat. Keeping clear weight transfers and always holding your upper body upright are other important principles. Start practicing your cat steps now!

chapter 4

Basic Hand Forms and Movement

Because tai chi is rooted in the Chinese martial art of boxing, understanding boxing hand forms and movement patterns will help you in learning tai chi. In this chapter, three key tai chi hand forms are introduced, and then eight major hand movement patterns and some exercises are introduced and illustrated. After familiarizing yourself with these exercises, you should be able to easily apply them to the tai chi forms starting in chapter 6 onward.

Hand Forms

The three major hand positions in tai chi are the fist, palm, and hook. As mentioned, hands in tai chi were used originally for various combat purposes; for example, the hook was used to hit an enemy's temple when the enemy was attacking from behind. When practiced for fitness, these forms help exercise the hand muscles and improve fine motor skills and function of the hands.

Fist

The fist is formed by bending all the fingers naturally into the palm of the hand with the thumb resting at the third joint of the index finger (see figure 4.1). Do not clench the fingers closed or together too firmly, and make sure the center of the palm is empty (i.e., there is space in the middle of your fist). Keep the fist straight with no angle from your wrist.

Common mistakes of the fist form are holding the fingers too tightly together (see figure 4.2a), putting the thumb inside the fist (see figure 4.2b), and bending the wrist too much (see figure 4.2c). Correct these mistakes by bending the fingers and holding them together slightly, always keeping the thumb outside the fist and resting on the index finger, and keeping the fist and forearm on the same line.

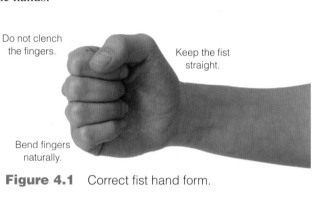

Do not clench the fingers.

Keep the fist straight.

Bend fingers naturally.

Figure 4.1   Correct fist hand form.

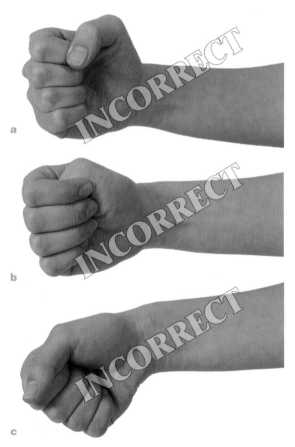

a

b

c

Figure 4.2   Incorrect fist hand forms: (a) fingers held too tightly together, (b) thumb inside the fist, and (c) angled wrist.

Palm

The palm is formed by bending the hand upward and holding all the fingers out in a natural, relaxed manner without them touching each other (see figure 4.3). The palm is vertical to the ground when used as a pushing palm (when the palm faces outward and moves away from the body); otherwise, it is perfectly fine to hold the palm facing outward and bent only slightly upward as long as it is in a natural position with the wrist and arm.

Common mistakes of the palm form are bending the fingers too much (see figure 4.4a), holding them too rigidly (see figure 4.4b), and pointing the fingertips out instead of in the upward vertical position for pushing hands (see figure 4.4c). Correct these mistakes by curving and relaxing the upper joints of the fingers naturally and holding them in place softly; keep about 90 degrees between the hand and forearm when doing a pushing hand.

Separate your fingers in a relaxed manner.

Bend your fingertips naturally.

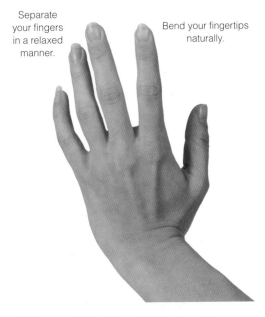

Figure 4.3   Correct palm hand form.

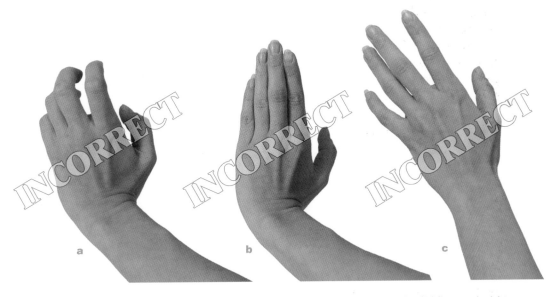

Figure 4.4   Incorrect palm hand forms: *(a)* fingers bent too much, *(b)* fingers held too rigid, and *(c)* fingertips pointed outward.

Hook

The hook is formed by touching all the fingertips and thumb together, with the wrist in a downward flexed position (see figure 4.5). Do not hold the fingers together too tightly; let them come together in a natural, relaxed manner.

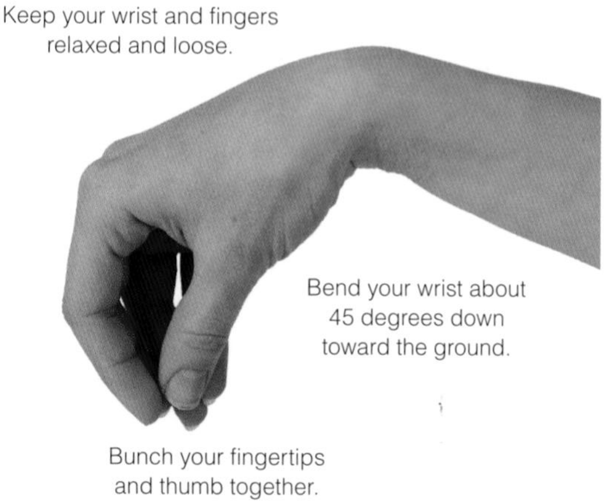

Keep your wrist and fingers relaxed and loose.

Bend your wrist about 45 degrees down toward the ground.

Bunch your fingertips and thumb together.

Figure 4.5 Correct hook hand form.

Common mistakes of the hook form are bending the wrist more than 45 degrees (see figure 4.6*a*), holding the wrist joint too rigidly (see figure 4.6*b*), and having the fingers too close to each other (see figure 4.6*c*). Correct these mistakes by bending the fingers naturally to keep a space inside the hand so that your fingers form a small cage and allowing your wrist joint to bend naturally.

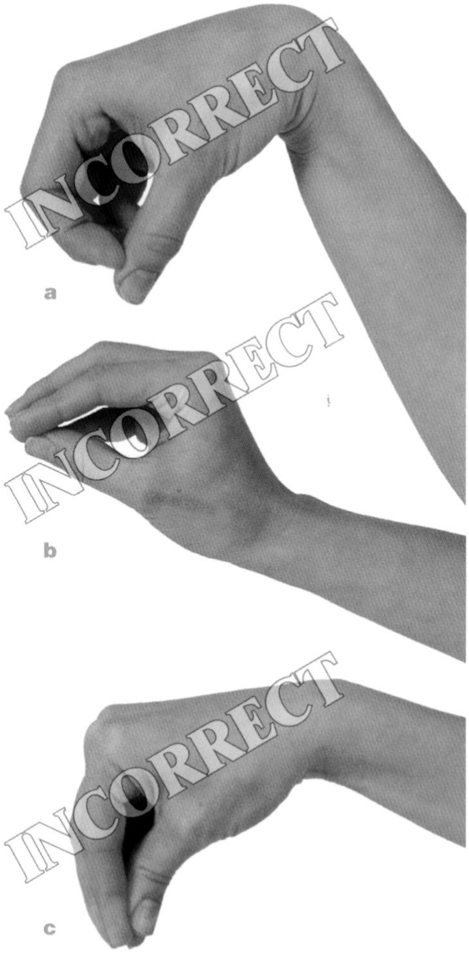

a

b

Figure 4.6 Incorrect hook hand forms: (*a*) wrist bent more than 45 degrees, (*b*) wrist held too rigidly, and (*c*) fingers too close to each other.

c

Hand Movement

Most tai chi hand movements are circular or curved; rarely does tai chi movement follow a straight line. The circular movement can be further divided into horizontal and vertical circles. The pattern of the hand movements can be a full circle, a half circle, an ellipse, or simply a curve. The movement of the two hands can be the opposite of each other, in the same direction, or in sequence with each other. Eight common hand movements are introduced in this section. You should be able to apply these movements to the tai chi forms that you will learn starting in chapter 6.

Vertical Circular Movement

In this movement, your hands make a full circle in front of your body. Movement path is summarized in figure 4.7. (Note: The solid line represents the right hand and arm, and the dotted line represents the left hand and arm. It is not a mirror representation; think of yourself as being behind the illustration.)

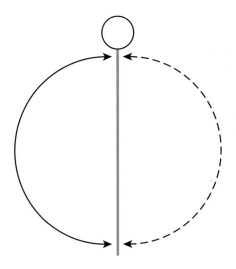

Figure 4.7 Movement path for Vertical Circular Movement.

(continued)

1 Stand at ease with the upper body held upright. Hold your hands open with fingers bent naturally. Cross your hands in front of your chest, with the left hand on the inside and both palms facing your chest. Relax your shoulders and breathe naturally.

2 Turn your left hand down and right hand up as the left hand moves upward and the right hand moves downward, ending in a holding-ball position with the left hand on top, right hand on the bottom, and palms facing each other. Keep your upper body upright. Relax your shoulders.

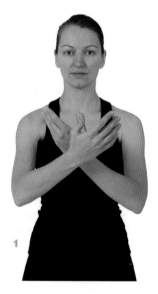

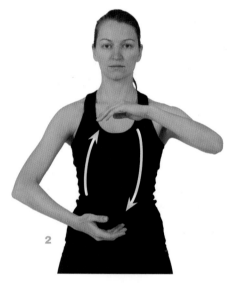

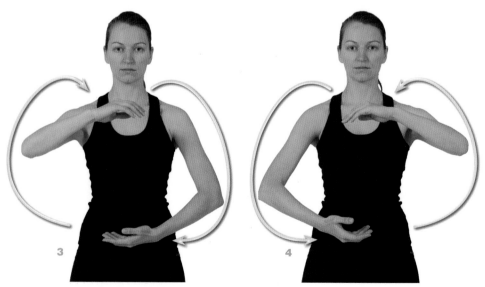

3 Move your arms and hands in opposite directions, with the left hand moving in a downward arc and the right hand moving in an upward arc counterclockwise, both simultaneously making a little over a half circle; end with the palms facing each other and your right hand on the top of the holding-ball position. Keep your upper body upright and relax your shoulders.

4 Moving back along the arc of the circular path performed previously, both arms and hands move clockwise in opposite directions, with the right hand moving downward and left hand moving upward simultaneously, stopping with palms facing each other in the holding-ball position with the left hand back at the top. Keep your upper body upright and relax your shoulders.

5 Repeat steps 2 and 3 several times.

Common mistakes of the Vertical Circular Movement are moving the arms and hands along an up-and-down straight line rather than an arc and not keeping the shoulders relaxed. Correct these mistakes by making sure your arm movement is curved, bending the arms throughout as if you were holding a big ball at all times, and keeping your upper body upright and your shoulders relaxed and down.

Inside Vertical Circular Movement in Sequence

In this movement, your hands move along two circles in front of your body, with the left hand moving clockwise and the right hand moving counterclockwise. In addition, as noted in the name of the movement, the left and right arms move in sequential order. Movement path is shown in figure 4.9. (Remember, the solid line represents the right hand and arm, and the dotted line represents the left hand and arm. It is not a mirror representation; think of yourself as being behind the illustration.)

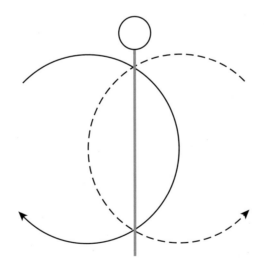

Figure 4.9 Movement path for Inside Vertical Circular Movement in Sequence.

(continued)

Inside Vertical Circular Movement in Sequence
(continued)

1 Extend your arms in front of your body in a relaxed, natural manner with about 45 degrees between your arms and body. Maintain about 5 inches (13 cm) of distance between your hands and body. Keep your upper body upright and relax your shoulders.

2 Move both arms along a full circle starting from the outer edge to the centerline of your body. The left arm moves along its full circle in a clockwise direction and the right arm moves counterclockwise for its full circle. To do this, start moving one arm along its own circle. The other arm starts once the first arm has made a half circle and is along the centerline of the body. The palm faces up when the hand is moving up and the palm faces the body when the hand is moving down. Be sure to keep about 5 inches (13 cm) between your hands and body. Keep your upper body upright and relax your shoulders.

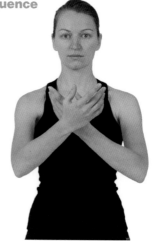

1

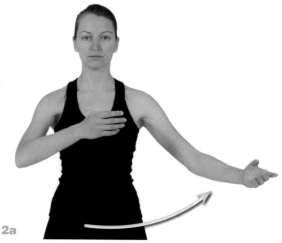

2a

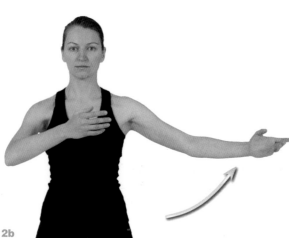

2b

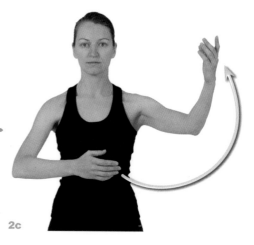

2c

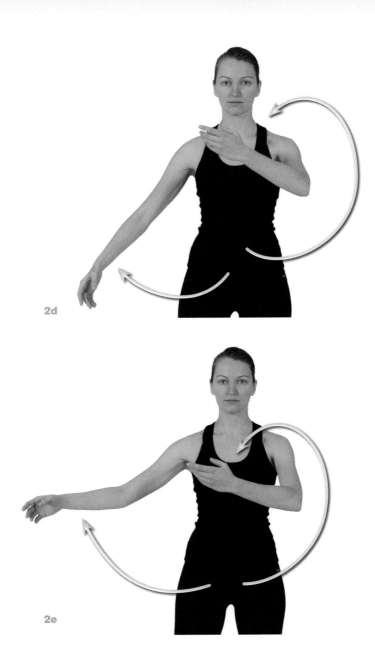

2d

2e

3 **Repeat the movements several times.**

Common mistakes of this hand movement are having tight shoulders; moving the arms or hands without making full, round circles; and moving the hands either too close or too far from the front of the body. Correct these mistakes by relaxing the shoulders, elbows, and wrists while moving; checking the paths of your hands by practicing in front of a mirror; and keeping your hands moving on a plane that is 5 inches (13 cm) away and parallel to the front of your body.

Outside Vertical Circular Movement in Sequence

In this movement, your hands also move along two circles in front of your body, but the right hand moves clockwise and the left hand moves counterclockwise. Again, as noted in the name of the movement, the left and right arms move in sequential order. Movement path is shown in figure 4.11. (The solid line represents the right hand and arm, and the dotted line represents the left hand and arm. It is not a mirror representation; think of yourself as being behind the illustration.)

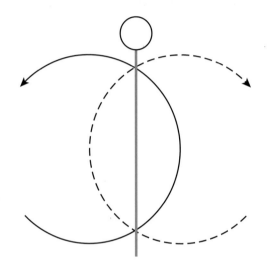

Figure 4.11   Movement path for Outside Vertical Circular Movement in Sequence.

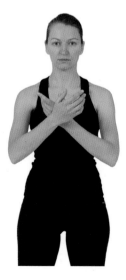

1 **Open your hands with fingers naturally bent and cross the hands in front of your chest, with the left hand on the inside and both palms facing your chest. Stand at ease with the upper body kept upright. Relax your shoulders and breathe naturally.**

2 Start moving your arm along its own circle, with one arm starting first and the other starting its path when the first arm is on the outer edge of the circle. To do this, the left hand and arm move upward while arcing away from the centerline of your body; then they move downward and upward again to the centerline of your body, making a full counterclockwise circle. The right hand and arm follow on their own clockwise circle once the left hand and arm have made a half circle. The palm faces up when the hand is moving up and it faces your body when the hand is moving down. Be sure to keep about 5 inches (13 cm) between your hands and body. Keep your upper body upright and relax your shoulders.

3 Repeat the movements several times.

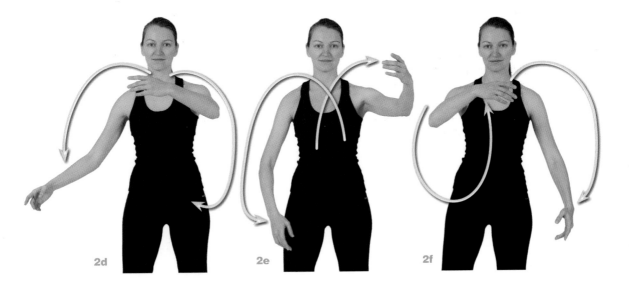

2a

2b

2c

2d

2e

2f

(continued)

Similar to the Inside Vertical Circular Movement in Sequence, common mistakes of this hand movement are holding the shoulders, arms, and hands too tightly; moving without making full, round circles; and moving the hands either too close or too far from the body. Correct these mistakes by relaxing your shoulders, elbows, and wrists while moving; checking the paths of your hands by practicing in front of a mirror; and keeping your hands moving within a plane that is 5 inches (13 cm) away and parallel to the front of your body.

Inside Vertical Circular Movement Together

In this movement, your hands once again move along two circles that are in front of your body, with the left hand moving clockwise and the right hand moving counterclockwise (i.e., moving from inside and down to outside and up). As noted in the name of the movement, the left and right arms move simultaneously along their opposite circular paths. Movement path is shown in figure 4.13. (The solid line represents the right hand and arm, and the dotted line represents the left hand and arm. It is not a mirror representation; think of yourself as being behind the illustration.)

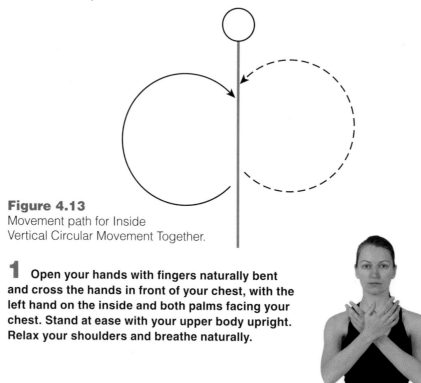

Figure 4.13
Movement path for Inside
Vertical Circular Movement Together.

1 **Open your hands with fingers naturally bent and cross the hands in front of your chest, with the left hand on the inside and both palms facing your chest. Stand at ease with your upper body upright. Relax your shoulders and breathe naturally.**

2 Keeping your upper body upright and shoulders relaxed, start moving both arms simultaneously down and then up along their own circular paths. The palms face up when the hands move up, and they face down when the hands move down. Keep about 5 inches (13 cm) of distance between your hands and your body.

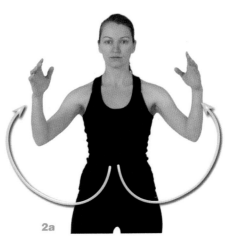

2a

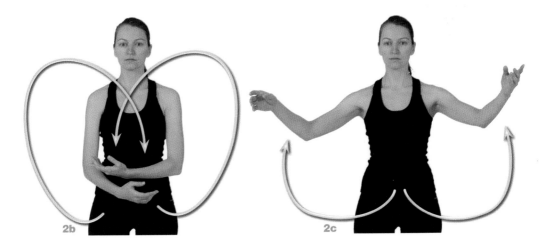

2b

2c

3 With your upper body upright and shoulders relaxed, keep moving your arms up along the circular paths, with the centers of the circles at about shoulder level. At the top of the circles, face the palms down. Keep about 5 inches (13 cm) of distance between your hands and your body.

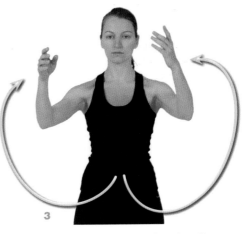

3

(continued)

4 Stop the movement when your hands return to the starting position in step 1. Be sure that your hands are open with fingers naturally bent. Relax your shoulders and breathe naturally.

5 Repeat the movement several times.

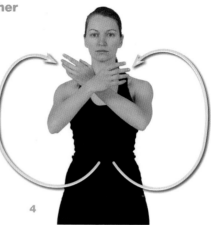

4

Similar to the Inside Vertical Circular Movement in Sequence described earlier, common mistakes of this hand movement are holding the shoulders, arms, and hands too tightly; moving without making full, round circles; moving the hands either too close or too far from the body; and holding the hands too high or too low when moving along the circular paths. Correct these mistakes by relaxing your shoulders, elbows, and wrists while moving; checking the paths of your hands by practicing in front of a mirror; keeping your hands moving on a plane about 5 inches (13 cm) away and parallel to your body; turning your palms as your arms and hands move (facing up when moving up and facing down or facing your body when moving down); and having the centers of the circles at shoulder level.

Outside Vertical Circular Movement Together

In this movement, your hands move along two circles that are in front of your body, with the right hand moving clockwise and left hand moving counterclockwise (i.e., moving from inside and up to outside and down). Both left and right arms move simultaneously along opposite circular paths. Movement path is shown in figure 4.15. (The solid line represents the right hand and arm, and the dotted line represents the left hand and arm. It is not a mirror representation; think of yourself as being behind the illustration.)

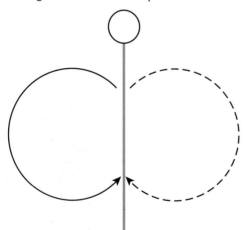

Figure 4.15   Movement path for Outside Vertical Circular Movement Together.

1 Open your hands with fingers naturally bent and cross the hands in front of your chest, with the left hand on the inside and both palms facing your chest. Stand at ease with your upper body upright. Relax your shoulders and breathe naturally.

2 Keeping your upper body upright and shoulders relaxed, start moving both arms up from the middle of your body and then down along their own circular paths. The palms face up when the hands move up and the palms face down when the hands move down. Keep about 5 inches (13 cm) of distance between your hands and your body.

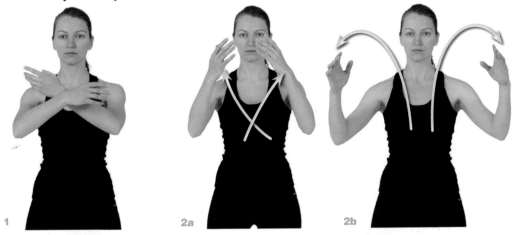

3 With your upper body upright and shoulders relaxed, keep moving your arms down along the circular paths, with the centers of the circles at about shoulder level. Face your palms down at the tops of the circles. Keep about 5 inches (13 cm) of distance between your hands and your body.

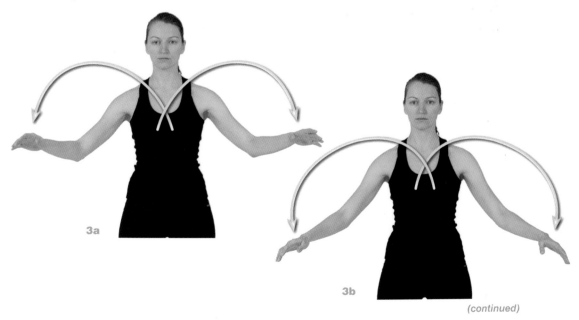

(continued)

4 Continue the movement along the circles and turn your palms up when your hands are along the midline of your body. Stop the movement when your hands return to the starting position in step 1. Be sure that the hands are open with fingers naturally bent. Relax your shoulders and breathe naturally.

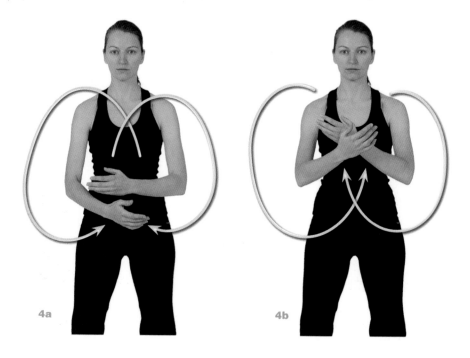

4a   4b

5 Repeat the movement several times.

Common mistakes of this hand movement are holding the shoulders, arms, and hands too tightly; moving without making full, round circles; moving the hands either too close or too far from the body; moving the hands too high or too low when moving along the circles; and moving the arms and hands in sequence rather than together. Correct these mistakes by relaxing your shoulders, elbows, and wrists while moving; checking the paths of your hands by practicing in front of a mirror; keeping your hands moving on a plane about 5 inches (13 cm) away and parallel to your body; turning your palms as your arms and hands move (facing up when moving up and facing down or facing your body when moving down); and making sure the centers of the circles are at shoulder level.

Horizontal Ellipse Movement in Sequence

In this movement, your hands move along a horizontal ellipse in front of your body. An ellipse is an oval that is symmetrical both horizontally and vertically. Both hands move in the same direction but in sequence, with the right hand on the top first moving clockwise and then the left hand moving clockwise, and then with the left hand on the top first moving counterclockwise and then the right hand moving counterclockwise. Movement path is shown in figure 4.17. (The solid line represents the right hand and arm, and the dotted line represents the left hand and arm. It is not a mirror representation; think of yourself as being behind the illustration.)

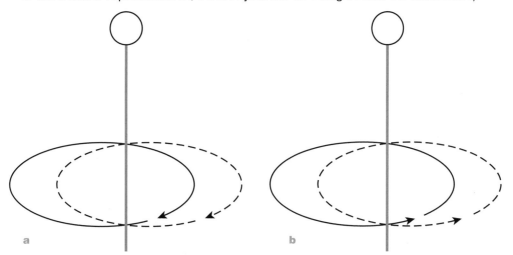

Figure 4.17 Movement path for Horizontal Ellipse Movement in Sequence: (*a*) clockwise and (*b*) counterclockwise.

1 Cross your hands and arms slightly in front of your chest with the right wrist on top of the left wrist and both palms up.

2 Stand at ease with your upper body upright and shoulders relaxed. Move your right hand back with the palm facing down and move your left hand forward with the palm facing up.

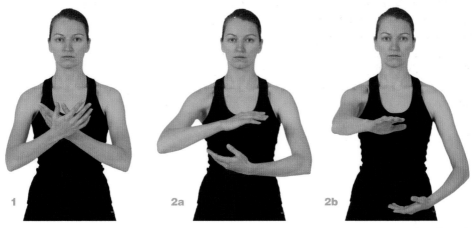

(continued)

3 Move your left hand forward while your right hand moves backward. Keep your left palm facing up and right palm facing down.

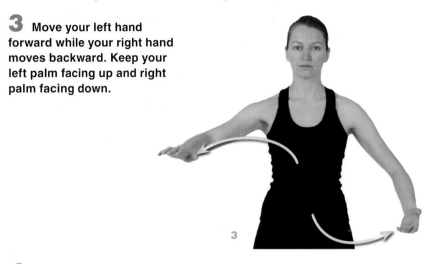

3

4 Keep both hands moving along their own ellipse. Start to move with your right hand forward, palm facing down, and turn your left hand over so the palm is facing the ground a bit at the front end of its ellipse; then gradually turn your left palm up again when moving your left hand back toward your body.

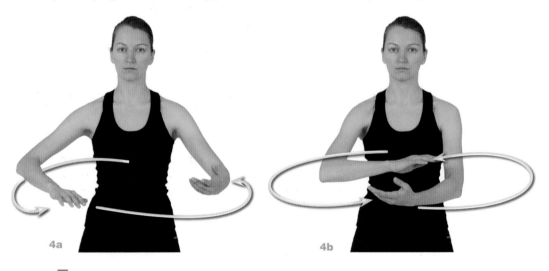

4a

4b

5 Repeat the movement several times. After you learn the movement, start with your left hand from the opposite direction, making horizontal counterclockwise ellipses.

Common mistakes of this hand movement are holding the shoulders, arms, and hands too tightly; moving without following the path of an ellipse; moving the hands either too close or too far from the front of the body; and having the palms facing the same direction. Correct these mistakes by relaxing your shoulders, elbows, and wrists while moving and by practicing in front of a mirror to check that your hands are moving along an elliptical path.

Vertical Ellipse Movement Together

In this movement, your hands move along a vertical ellipse in front of your body. Both hands move together in the same direction: counterclockwise first (down from right shoulder to left hip and then up) and then clockwise (down from left shoulder to right hip). Movement path is shown in figure 4.19. (The solid line represents the right hand and arm, and the dotted line represents the left hand and arm. It is not a mirror representation; think of yourself as being behind the illustration.)

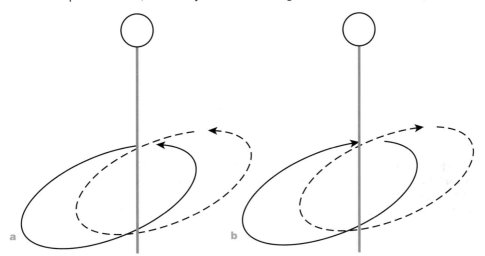

Figure 4.19 Movement path for Vertical Ellipse Movement Together: (*a*) counterclockwise and (*b*) clockwise.

1 **Stand at ease with your upper body upright. With open hands and fingers naturally bent, cross your hands in front of your chest, with the left hand on the inside and both palms facing your chest. Relax your shoulders and breathe naturally.**

2 **With your shoulders relaxed, separate your hands and move the right hand to the right and turn the palm down; at the same time, turn the left palm down. Both hands are at the top of the vertical ellipse now. While doing this movement, turn**

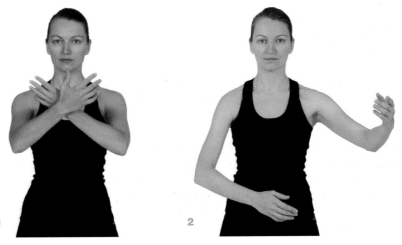

(continued)

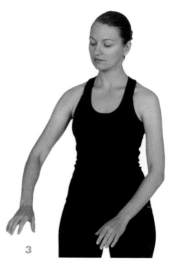

your head slightly to the right, with your eyes and face following the movement of your hands. At the bottom of the vertical ellipse, both hands move up.

3 With your upper body upright and shoulders relaxed, keep your hands moving. Both palms turn to face toward your body and your head and eyes follow the movement of your hands.

4 With your upper body upright and shoulders and elbows relaxed, keep moving both hands up along their own ellipses, and turn both palms up when the hands are moving up.

5 Repeat the movement by moving both hands down following the same elliptical path. The right palm turns up naturally when right hand moves down; turn the palm down after your front arm and upper arm reach about 90 degrees. Keep your palms turned down as soon as your hands start to move down.

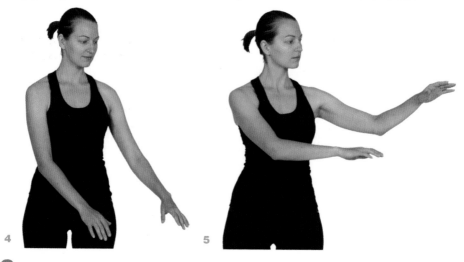

6 Repeat the movement several times. After you learn the movement, change it to the opposite direction, making a clockwise vertical ellipse.

Common mistakes of this hand movement are holding the shoulders, arms, and hands too tightly; moving without following the path of an ellipse; moving the hands either too close to or too far from the front of the body; moving the hands too high or low; and not following the hand movements with the head and eyes. Correct these mistakes by relaxing your shoulders, elbows, and wrists while moving; checking the paths of your hands by practicing in front of a mirror; keeping your hands moving within the ellipse surface of about 5 inches (13 cm) in front of your body; and letting your head and eyes follow the movement of your hands.

Back-and-Forth Vertical Side Ellipse Movement in Sequence

In this movement, your hand moves along an ellipse on one side of your body. Practice the other side after repeating the movement on one side several times. Movement path is shown in figure 4.21. (The solid line represents the right hand and arm, and the dotted line represents the left hand and arm. It is not a mirror representation; think of yourself as being behind the illustration.)

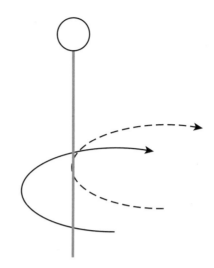

Figure 4.21   Movement path for Back-and-Forth Vertical Side Ellipse Movement in Sequence.

1 Stand at ease with your upper body upright and shoulders relaxed. With your hands open and fingers naturally bent, cross both hands in front of your body, with the left hand on the inside. Breathe naturally.

2 Separate your hands by moving the left hand down along a side ellipse on the left side of your body, palm facing up. Keep your right hand as the front hand, remaining in starting position. Shoulders are relaxed.

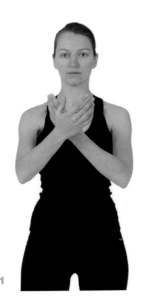

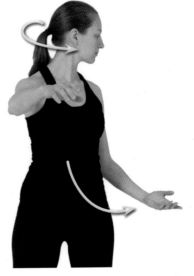

(continued)

3 Raise your left hand with the fingertips up and palm facing out to the front. Move your right hand down a little in front of your chest. Turn your body slightly to the left. Shoulders are relaxed.

4 Keep moving the left hand up along the path of the ellipse and turn your body back to facing the front. Relax your shoulders and elbows.

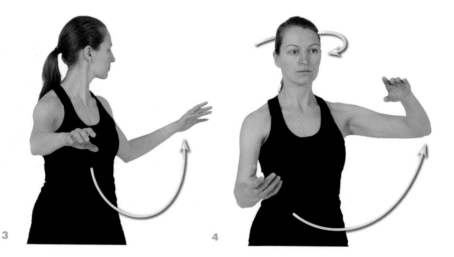

3

4

5 Repeat the movement several times. After you learn the movement for the left hand and arm, practice the movement with the right hand and arm on the right side of body.

Common mistakes of this hand movement are holding the shoulders, arms, and hands too tightly; moving without following the path of an ellipse; moving the hands too high or too low; and not following the hand movements with the upper body. Correct these mistakes by relaxing your shoulders, elbows, and wrists while moving; checking the paths of your hands by practicing in front of a mirror; and keeping your hands moving along the ellipse's plane and letting your upper body turn to follow hand movements naturally.

By learning and practicing these hand positions and movements, you will become familiar with core tai chi movements and related movement patterns. They are not actually tai chi techniques, but you should start to enjoy the feeling you will likely experience doing these tai chi–related movements. Building on these basic movements, you will start to learn specific tai chi forms and corresponding moves starting in chapter 6, and you will be able to integrate them naturally into the forms. Start practicing and enjoying these movements!

chapter 5

Basic Stances

Zhan zhuan is a term used widely in all forms of Chinese martial arts and mind–body exercises. *Zhan* means "stand" and *zhuan* means "post." Together, these two characters mean "stand like a post," or simply, "stance."

When practicing your stance, you stand with the required posture for some time. Stance is often compared to the foundation of a building. You need a strong and solid foundation to be able to construct a tall building. It is so important that there is a well-known Chinese saying reflecting its significance: "Without practicing stance, one learns nothing (from martial arts or mind–body exercise) over time." According to Chinese medicine, certain meridians are stimulated in specific stances. As a result, qi or vital energy related to these meridians is promoted. The importance of stance is also supported in modern exercise physiology research. Studies have shown that many muscle groups are involved in stance practice. Because the load comes from the weight of the body, the training dose can be easily controlled and adjusted (e.g., bending the knees more to increase the intensity).

Furthermore, because the muscles are isometrically trained, stance is effective in increasing leg muscle mass and strength in a time-efficient manner. Stance is also excellent for meditation. After some stance practice, you should feel a sense of relaxation and peace in your mind, which is why the stance is often called *standing meditation* in China. However, do not force yourself to meditate when you start stance practice. Stance practice can be boring and hard work when you start, thus making it hard to meditate at first. It is fine to let your mind wander as you practice. When you practice at home, you are encouraged to listen to music. You will find yourself able to meditate easily and naturally after several weeks of stance practice.

TIP When done correctly, regular stance practice can help improve your emotional state and prevent certain health problems, such as headaches and colds. Yet even with its benefits, you should not do stance practice when you are sad, you are very sick, or you have just eaten a large meal or consumed alcohol. In these situations, stance practice is not beneficial.

As it is in other martial arts and mind–body exercises, stance is an essential part of tai chi training, and this chapter introduces a few common practice stances. Because these stances were designed specifically for tai chi, they are sometimes called the *tai chi stances*. By practicing stances regularly, especially when starting to learn tai chi, you strengthen your legs, which will give you better control of your balance and movement, thus making it easier to meditate. As a result, you will learn tai chi faster and it will be more enjoyable. However, do not expect quick results. Usually it takes two to three months before you start to feel the benefits of stance practice. Consistency is crucial in stance practice. Some tai chi masters compare stance practice to recharging a battery—after recharging, a depleted battery becomes filled with new energy and life. Stance practice will infuse your body with new energy, leading to faster recovery, but this will take time to achieve.

TIP Control the intensity of the stance with appropriate knee bending; the more bent the knees are, the higher the intensity. Start with slightly bent knees and gradually increase the degree of bending. Hold your upper body upright, because qi (life energy) may not flow well if your upper body is inclined too far forward or backward.

Try to do stance practice 20 to 30 minutes every day even if you do not practice any other tai chi forms or routines. Stance practice requires little space and can take place almost anywhere, so reaching a daily goal of 20 to 30 minutes should not be difficult. Try to integrate stance practice into your daily life, such as during breaks, while waiting at the bus stop, and so on. In this way, practice becomes a way to energize yourself during downtime rather than a burden on your time. Also, it may be helpful to do stance practice with others. Good social support will make stance practice easier and more fun. In addition, practicing together can significantly improve the efficiency of your practice because of the qi field created by a group of people practicing together.

Being able to relax during stance practice is difficult yet important. To achieve this, your mind should be relaxed first. After overcoming the first stages of muscle strength and endurance challenges, you should start to learn how to relax. Using your imagination during practice could be helpful, such as imagining warm water flowing slowly from your head to your shoulders, arms, legs, and feet.

Wuji Stance

Recall that chapter 1 introduced the wuji diagram (see figure 1.4 on page 8) as simply a circle. The circle represents the original state of the universe, in which everything was static. The wuji stance somewhat reflects this static meaning.

During wuji stance practice, stand in a natural manner with legs shoulder-width apart and knees slightly bent. Relax your mind and start to meditate. Breathe naturally with the Dan Tian relaxed. As discussed earlier, the Dan Tian is located in your front lower belly. Maintain the stance for 5 to 10 minutes. It is okay to adjust the distance between your legs for comfort. To help relax and meditate, you can also think through each part of your body based on the earlier description of the correct tai chi postures and adjust your body accordingly.

1 Stand relaxed with your legs shoulder-width apart, keeping your body weight equally divided between both legs (see figures for a side view and front view). Relax your upper body, keeping it upright, and relax your shoulders. Hold your chin steady, with your eyes looking forward. Breathe naturally with your Dan Tian area relaxed.

2 Bend your knees slightly, but keep your upper body upright in the same vertical line.

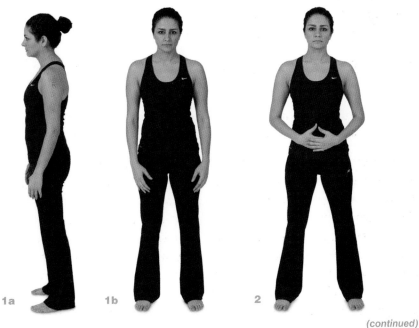

1a   1b   2

(continued)

Common mistakes in the wuji stance include distributing body weight unevenly onto the legs, bending the upper body forward or backward too much, having straight knees, and not relaxing the body. Correct these mistakes by distributing body weight equally between both legs, keeping your whole body upright but relaxed, and breathing naturally.

Circle Stance

This stance is named for the shape that the arms hold, which is a circle. In this stance, you stand with your legs apart and knees bent, and you form an open circle with your arms in front of your body, with the palms facing each other or angled slightly down toward the Dan Tian. Hold this stance for 3 to 5 minutes and repeat it two to five times, with 5-minute breaks in between.

TIP Make sure your whole body feels as one. In circle stance, for example, rather than feeling your arms and legs separately, you should feel as if you were going to hug someone using your whole body.

1 Stand with your legs about shoulder-width apart and keep your body weight divided equally between both legs. Your knees should be bent (slightly at first, but increase the bend as your legs get stronger). Using your arms, form a circle in front of your body. Relax your upper body, keeping it upright, and relax your shoulders. Hold your chin steady, with your eyes looking forward. Breathe naturally with the Dan Tian area relaxed.

2 Bend both knees, keeping the upper body upright in the same vertical line, and relax your shoulders (see figures for a front and side view). Keep an angle of about 45 degrees between your upper arms and upper body. Keep an angle of about 5 to 10 degrees between the forearms and upper arms.

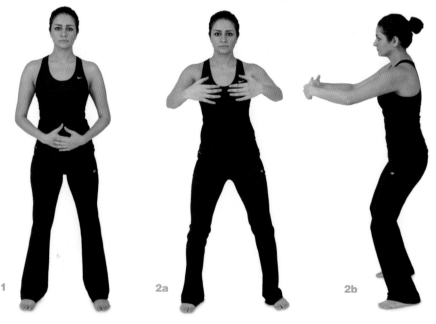

1   2a   2b

Common mistakes in the circle stance include standing with the legs too close to each other, bending too little or too much, leaning the upper body forward or backward too much, holding the arms too high or too low, and not relaxing the shoulders. Correct these mistakes by separating your legs and distributing your body weight equally between both legs; keeping your whole body upright but relaxed, especially the shoulders; bending your knees at a comfortable angle initially; gradually increasing the bend in your knees; and breathing naturally.

Open–Close Stance

This stance is named for the variation in how the arms are held (i.e., a combination of opened and closed). During the practice, you start in the circle stance position with legs apart, knees bent, and arms in front in a circle. Open your arms slowly until they are at a 45-degree angle from the body, and then close your arms slowly, ending with your hands joined in front of the Dan Tian. Breathe in when your arms are opening and breathe out when they are closing. Breathe in a deep, slow, and relaxed manner at the same speed throughout the opening and closing phases. Repeat 8 to 12 times. The eyes can be slightly closed. Enjoy the relaxed feeling this movement provides.

1 **Stand with your legs about shoulder-width apart, body weight evenly distributed between both legs, and knees bent. Form a circle using both arms in front of your body, keeping an angle of about 45 degrees between your upper arms and upper body and an angle of 5 to 10 degrees between the forearms and upper arms. Relax your upper body, keeping it upright, and relax your shoulders. Hold your chin steady, with eyes looking forward (eyes can be closed after learning the movement). Breathe naturally.**

2 **Keep your body weight evenly distributed between both legs and bend your knees. Open both arms, with the upper arms parallel to the ground and at an angle of 45 degrees to the front of your body. Breathe in when your arms are opening.**

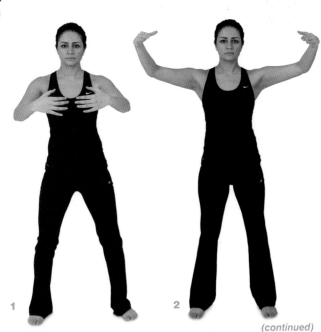

1

2

(continued)

3 With both knees still bent, keep the upper body upright and shoulders relaxed. Return your arms to the starting position, continuing to step 4. Breathe out when your arms are closing.

4 With the knees still bent and shoulders relaxed, move both arms back and down toward the Dan Tian. Stop with your left hand (if you are male) or right hand (if you are female) slightly touching the Dan Tian and the palm of your right hand (males) or left hand (females) touching the back of your left hand (males) or right hand (females). Breathe naturally and focus your mind on the Dan Tian, where you should feel warmth as your skill level improves.

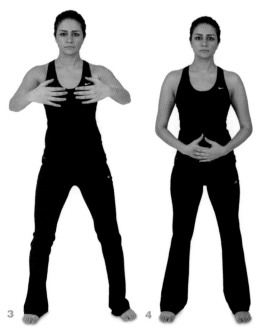

Common mistakes in the open–close stance include standing with the legs too close to each other, bending the knees too little or too much, leaning the upper body forward or backward too much, holding the arms too high or too low, not relaxing the shoulders, straightening the knees when opening the arms, and not coordinating breathing with arm movements. Correct these mistakes by separating your legs and distributing your body weight equally between both legs; keeping your whole body upright but relaxed, especially the shoulders; bending your knees comfortably and increasing the bend gradually; keeping the same degree of bending when your arms open and close; and breathing in while your arms open and breathing out while they close.

Up–Down Stance

This stance is named for its variation in leg movements (i.e., a combination of straight and bent legs). During the practice, you stand with legs shoulder-width apart and raise both arms slowly to the same level as your shoulders. Squat down slowly as your arms move down with the wrists slightly bent, and then return to the original starting position. You breathe in when your arms move up and breathe out when they move down. Breathe in a slow and relaxed manner. Repeat 8 to 12 times. Close your eyes slightly after becoming familiar with the stance and enjoy the relaxed feeling the movement provides.

1 With your upper body upright, stand with both legs straight, about shoulder-width apart, with body weight evenly distributed between both. Raise both arms in front of your body to shoulder level. Breathe in when your arms move up.

2 Keeping your upper body upright, slowly bend your knees while moving your arms down (see figures for a front view and side view). Breathe out when your arms move down. Hold the squat position for 10 to 15 seconds (hold longer as you get stronger), and then stand up, returning to the starting position shown in step 1.

1

2a

2b

Common mistakes in the up–down stance include standing with the legs too close to each other, leaning the upper body forward or backward too much, holding the arms too high or too low, bending the knees, and not coordinating breathing with arm movements. Correct these mistakes by separating your legs and distributing your body weight evenly between both legs, keeping your whole body upright but relaxed, coordinating your arm movements, bending your knees, and breathing.

Loose–Firm Stance

This stance is named for the contrast of the exercise load on the arms and legs (i.e., a combination of on and off loads on the arms and legs). Start by standing with your legs naturally apart, knees slightly bent. Shift your body weight to your left leg while you raise your body slightly (knees are still bent and arms are open outward), and continue shifting your body weight onto your left leg while moving your curved arms down and turning your body 45 degrees to the right. Finish shifting your body weight onto your left leg with your arms held in front of your body and your right heel touching the ground. Your left leg is firm while your right leg is loose in this movement. Repeat steps 1 through 5 (listed next) by moving your body weight back onto both legs first and then transferring your body weight onto your right leg, remembering to end the stance with your arms in front of your body while your body weight is on your right leg and your left heel is touching the ground. Now your right leg is firm while your left leg is loose. Repeat the movement (switching from left to right leg) three to four times. End your practice by turning your body to the front, with your body weight evenly distributed between both legs. Arms move down to return to the original standing position.

(continued)

1 With the upper body upright, stand with your legs straight and about shoulder-width apart, with body weight evenly distributed between both. Raise both arms in front of your body to shoulder level. Breathe in when the arms move up.

2 Keeping the upper body upright, slowly bend your knees and move your arms down at the same time. Breathe out while you do this movement and breathe in when you are in a squatting position.

3 With your upper body still upright, continue shifting your body weight onto your left leg as you turn your body 45 degrees to the right. Move your curved arms down.

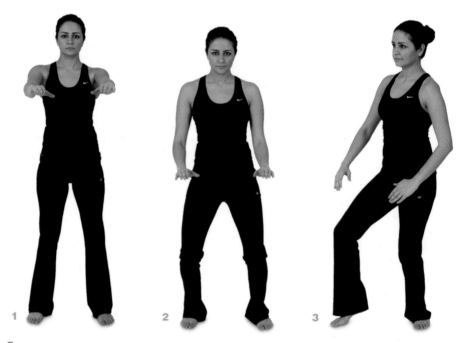

4 For a loose right side, keep your upper body upright and start to shift your body weight onto your left leg while your body rises slightly with the knees still bent. Open your arms outward at the same time.

5 When the body weight is completely shifted, your arms held out in front of your upper body. Raise your right toes and place your right heel on the ground to form a right empty step (your left leg is firm while your right leg is loose when the movement is completed). Raise your right hand in a curve to nose level, with the palm facing left and your right elbow slightly bent. The left hand moves down and back until it reaches the level of your right elbow, palm facing to the right.

6 For the left side, keeping the upper body upright and knees bent, start to transfer body weight onto your right leg while you raise your body slightly. Open your arms outward.

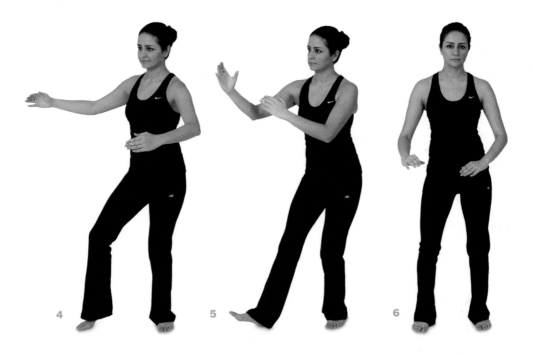

7 Keeping the upper body upright, continue shifting your body weight onto your right leg as you turn your body 45 degrees to the left. Move your curved arms downward.

8 When the body weight is completely shifted, your arms are held out in front of your upper body. Raise your left toes and touch your left heel on the ground to form a left empty step (your right leg now is firm while your left leg is loose when the movement is completed). Raise your left hand in a curve to nose level, with your palm facing to the right and elbow slightly bent. The right hand moves down and back until it reaches the level of your left elbow, palm facing left.

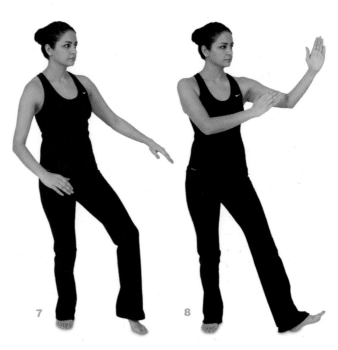

(continued)

9 To end the movement, start to transfer your body weight toward the front and return your body weight equally to both legs. At the same time, move your arms to the front.

10 Keeping your upper body upright and body weight evenly distributed between both legs, straighten your legs, which are shoulder-width apart. Return both arms to the front of your body at shoulder level.

11 Lower your arms to return to the starting position. Stand naturally and relaxed.

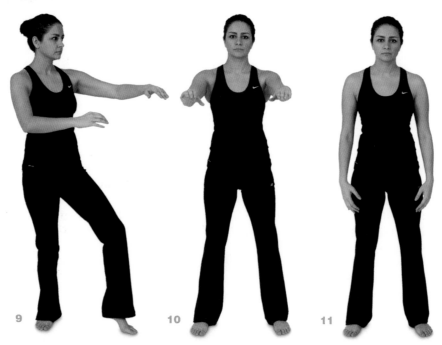

Common mistakes in the loose–firm stance include not clearly transferring weight between the legs, leaning the upper body forward or backward too much, not relaxing the shoulders, and not coordinating the turning body, bending knee, and moving arms. Correct these mistakes by slowly but clearly transferring your body weight during left and right stances, and make sure one leg is firm and the other one is empty when completing the stance. Keep your upper body upright.

Yin–Yang Stance

As introduced earlier, the yin–yang concept is the foundation of tai chi movement. This stance is named *yin–yang* because the body weight shifts between the legs from emptiness or looseness (yin) to firmness (yang). Start this stance with your legs naturally apart and raise both arms slowly to shoulder level, similar to the beginning of the up–down stance. Arc your right arm downward while shifting your body weight onto your left leg. End with your arms and hands positioned as if holding a large ball in front of the left side of your body and with your body weight fully on your left leg and your right toes touching the ground. Repeat steps 1 through 3 (listed next), but this time shift your body weight onto your right leg and arc your left arm downward. End as if you were holding a large ball in front of your right side, with your body weight fully on your right leg and your left toes touching the ground. End the practice by returning your body weight equally onto both legs. Bring your arms down to the starting standing position.

1 With the upper body upright and body weight evenly divided between both legs, stand with your legs straight about shoulder-width apart. Raise both arms in front of your body to shoulder level. Breathe in when moving your arms up.

2 For the left-leg stance, lift your right heel while keeping your toes on the ground and rotate your foot out about 45 degrees while at the same time turning your upper body slightly to the left, using your waist as the axis. Put your right heel back down on the ground. Move your body weight onto the left leg at the same time, move both arms down 3 to 4 inches (8-10 cm), and bend your elbows so that there is about a 5-degree angle with your forearms instead of holding your arms out straight; keep your left palm facing down. Arc your right arm downward and then toward your left side at the same time as you turn the upper body.

3 Keeping your upper body upright, complete the transfer of body weight onto your left leg and put your heel down. Move your right foot to the inner side of your left foot, with the right toes slightly touching the ground. Stop moving your right hand when it is under your left hand, palms facing each other (as if holding a ball on the left side of your body).

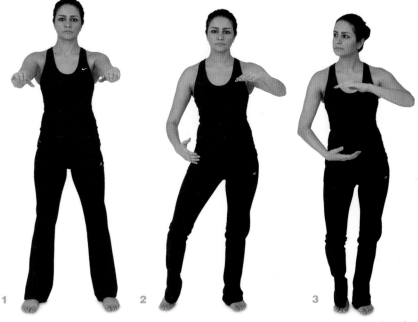

(continued)

4 For the right-leg stance, separate your legs by returning your right foot to its original position, toes turning out about 45 degrees, while also turning your upper body slightly to the right. Start to move your body weight onto your right leg. Move your right arm back along its arc path to its original position.

5 Keep transferring your body weight onto your right leg while moving your right arm up with the palm facing down. Move your left arm down, following the same arc of the right arm. Lift the heel of your left foot off the ground.

6 Keeping your upper body upright, complete the transfer of body weight to your right leg and move your left foot to the inside of the right foot, with your left toes slightly touching the ground. Stop moving your left hand when it is under your right hand, palms facing each other (as if holding a ball on the right side of your body).

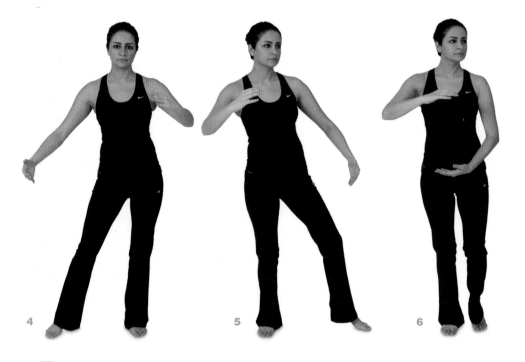

4   5   6

7 Repeat the left and right yin–yang stance several times.

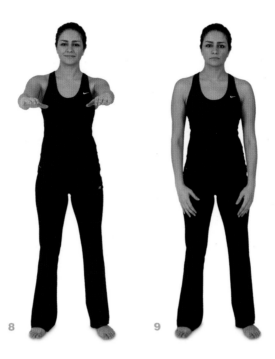

8 To end the movement, keep your upper body upright and start to return your body to face the front while returning your weight evenly to both legs. Return both arms out in front of your body at shoulder level.

9 Move both arms down, stand upright, and return to the starting position.

Common mistakes of the yin–yang stance include not clearly transferring weight between the legs, leaning the upper body forward or backward too much, not coordinating the bending knees and moving arms, and not moving the arms in smooth arcs. Correct these mistakes by slowly but clearly transferring body weight when forming left and right stances, making sure one leg is firm and the other one is empty when completing the stance on one side, keeping the upper body upright, and moving your arms in smooth arcs.

After learning tai chi stances, you have learned all the basic movements of tai chi and now have a solid foundation of tai chi. Starting with the next chapter, you will learn tai chi forms and be able to experience and enjoy the flow of tai chi. Meanwhile, keep practicing all basics learned since they will help improve your forms and routines practice.

part II

Tai Chi Forms

Often people just starting to learn tai chi are expected to jump right into the routines using as many as 108 forms. As a result, beginners are often confused and discouraged by the complexity of the instructions along with the skills required. The routines, in fact, consist of many single forms, which can be learned much more easily individually. By learning these forms individually, you as a beginner can memorize the movements quickly and start to understand the principles of tai chi. More important, you will be able to enjoy the related health benefits immediately.

In chapters 6 to 9, you will learn 14 popular forms used in tai chi. To help you more readily enjoy the health benefits, we have organized the forms according to their key functions or contributions to health: cardiovascular health in chapter 6, stress management and low-back heath in chapter 7, balance in chapter 8, and coordination in chapter 9. To help you as a beginner learn and remember a form and its movement, Chinese tai chi masters created names for each form. Some forms are named after animals; other forms are named for the characteristics of the movements. For each form, its name in Chinese spelling, including its Chinese characters, appears along with its English translation and a short explanation. Then, in a step-by-step manner, movements from starting position through transition to closing position are presented. Some key callouts for each movement are also provided with each illustration. After you learn movements individually, all those movement illustrations are then presented together in sequence to help you connect the movements together. Finally, some tips on best practice for each form are included at the end of each form's description.

chapter 6

Forms for Cardiovascular Health

Cardiovascular disease is a major cause of illness and the leading cause of death for both men and women in the United States. A sedentary lifestyle is an important modifiable risk factor for cardiovascular disease. Physical activity has been proven to provide a number of cardiovascular benefits, and a physically active lifestyle has been shown to reduce cardiovascular disease risks by 35 to 55 percent. In this chapter, after a brief introduction of the cardiovascular system and how it can benefit from physical activity and tai chi, you will learn three popular single forms that are beneficial for the cardiovascular system. Large arm movement is one of the beneficial characteristics of these forms. In addition to the positive effects on the arms themselves, these movements also engage the upper-back muscles so that they are actively used in this practice, resulting in a positive impact on the cardiovascular system. More important, according to TCM the three heart- and lung-related meridians are distributed in the arms. The flow of qi along these meridians is helped by moving the arms regularly, thus helping to improve cardiovascular health.

The cardiovascular system consists of the heart and blood vessels (arteries, veins, and capillaries). It transports oxygen to the muscles and organs and removes waste products, including carbon dioxide. The arteries carry blood from the heart to the body, and the veins carry blood back to the heart. Regular physical activity is essential to keep the cardiovascular system functioning well. Unfortunately, many Americans live a sedentary lifestyle, and as a result, one in three American adults has some form of cardiovascular disease. Cardiovascular disease is the leading cause of death in not only the United States but also the world. It can increase the risk of heart attack, heart failure, sudden death, stroke, and cardiac rhythm problems, thus resulting in decreased quality of life and life expectancy. Risk factors that can be prevented or treated include high blood pressure, high cholesterol, excess weight, physical inactivity, smoking, diabetes, excessive alcohol consumption, illegal drug use, and stress.

Besides smoking, physical inactivity is perhaps the most important behavioral risk factor because it is often the cause of other risk factors, including high blood pressure, high cholesterol, excess weight, and diabetes. In addition, physical activity can help reduce stress. If you regularly participate in aerobic exercise such as walking, swimming, running, or bicycling, you are improving your cardiovascular system. Known benefits of regular aerobic exercise include improved lung and heart strength, reduced blood levels of harmful LDL cholesterol, increased blood levels of helpful HDL cholesterol, increased physical and mental stamina, and reduced risk of chronic diseases such as heart disease, stroke, and type 2 diabetes. These positive changes from exercise significantly reduce the risk of getting cardiovascular disease.

So, what about tai chi? Can doing tai chi help your cardiovascular system and thus help prevent cardiovascular disease? The answer is yes! Tai chi has many cardiovascular benefits. First, it is a light- to moderate-intensity aerobic exercise. People with cardiovascular disease can practice hand movements, leg movements, and stance separately so that exercise intensity can be controlled at a low to light level. In contrast, a significant cardiorespiratory workout can be achieved by deeply bending the knees throughout a full tai chi routine. Second, tai chi practice is safe as a means of exercise therapy. No negative or adverse effects have been reported, according to a review of tai chi–based clinical trials. Third, tai chi brings a meditative aspect to its practice, thus fostering stress reduction. Finally, it helps promote the circulation of qi along the meridians that are directly responsible for cardiovascular health, according to TCM theory.

Many cardiologists prescribe tai chi as an adjunct therapy for treatment of heart problems or as preventative therapy. According to several systematic reviews published in medical literature, tai chi has already been shown to be a safe and beneficial therapy for some patients with cardiovascular disease. In this chapter, you will learn three popular tai chi forms, all of which can benefit your cardiovascular system.

You can practice these forms independently or integrate them into other exercise routines or programs, such as in your warm-up or cool-down. Practice tai chi to make your heart healthier!

TIP A typical exercise routine should include a warm-up (3-5 minutes), exercise (at least 20 minutes), and cool-down (5-10 minutes). Make sure you do not stop movement suddenly. Stop movement only after your heart rate slows down, you are breathing easily, and you can carry on a conversation without difficulty.

Level
- ▶ Beginner

Benefits
- ▶ Strengthens the upper body.
- ▶ Strengthens the legs.
- ▶ Improves the cardiovascular system.
- ▶ Improves body awareness.
- ▶ Improves qi flow.

Contraindications
- ▶ Falling with loss of balance

Parting Mustang's Mane

Ye Ma Fen Zong

The Chinese name of this form, *Ye Ma Fen Zong*, derives from its movements. The movements are similar to those of a mustang's mane while running (i.e., one arm raises while the other arm lowers, like an undulating horse's mane, as body weight shifts from one leg to the other). According to TCM, six major meridians pass through the arms and are activated during this form. As a result, qi flow along these meridians is promoted. For better health benefits, consider focusing your mind on the Dan Tian (the lower part of the belly) during practice.

TIP All movements are coordinated with each other (i.e., simultaneously shift body weight slowly from one leg to the other and move the arms gradually).

1 **For the starting position, stand with your legs naturally shoulder-width apart and with your feet parallel to each other. Keep your upper body, head, and neck upright. Hold your chin slightly down and relax your face with a slight smile. Hang your arms down along your sides with your hands naturally resting beside your thighs. Keep your body weight equally distributed between both legs. Clear your mind and keep a peaceful mental state throughout the whole form.**

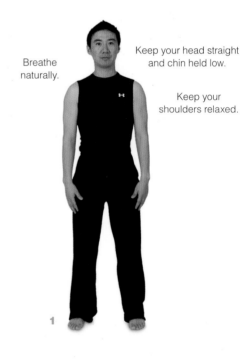

Keep your head straight and chin held low.

Breathe naturally.

Keep your shoulders relaxed.

2 Raise your arms slowly in front of your body until they are level with your shoulders. Your arms will be parallel to each other, shoulder-width apart, and your palms will be facing down. Keep your upper body, head, and neck upright. Hold your chin slightly down and relax your face with a slight smile. Keep your body weight distributed equally between both legs.

Breathe in while your arms move up.

Hold your head high and facing forward with the chin slightly down.

Do not bend your wrists.

Keep your head straight.

Keep your upper body straight.

Do not squat so far that your knees go past your toes.

3 For Parting Mustang's Mane (Left), slowly squat while you move both arms down simultaneously to the level of your waist. Keep your upper body upright while squatting. Note that *Left* or *Right* refers to the front leg when a Parting Mustang's Mane movement is finished. Parting Mustang's Mane (Left), therefore, means that the Parting Mustang's Mane movement finishes with the left leg in front.

Relax both shoulders.

4 Move your body weight onto your right leg. Raise your left leg slightly and move it closer to your right foot, with only your left toes touching the ground; meanwhile, move your right arm up and your left arm down, moving them along a circle. End with both hands in front of you as if you were holding a large ball.

End with all body weight on the right leg.

(continued)

5 Raise your left leg and take a full step out to the side, with your left heel touching the ground and your left toes pointing straight out to the left. Raise your left arm and cross both arms in front of your chest.

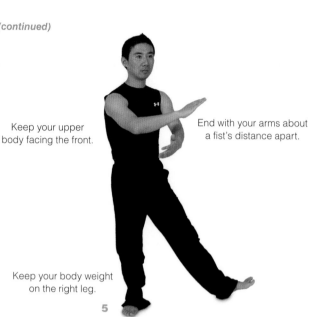

Keep your upper body facing the front.

End with your arms about a fist's distance apart.

Keep your body weight on the right leg.

5

6 To complete Parting Mustang's Mane (Left), turn your upper body to the left and shift your body weight gradually onto your left leg while your right hand moves down and your left hand moves slightly up. End the move with your legs in a left bow step (learned in chapter 3), right arm slightly in front of your upper body and right hand down alongside your right hip, left palm open toward your face. To maintain stability, both heels should be on parallel lines with about a foot (30 cm) between them. Make sure there is about a foot (30 cm) between your feet when in a bow step, and make sure your front foot is perpendicular to the body.

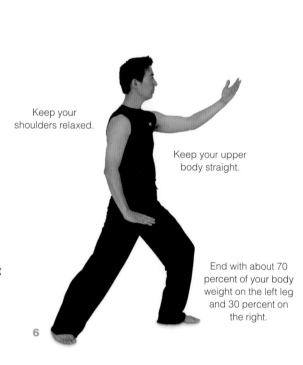

Keep your shoulders relaxed.

Keep your upper body straight.

End with about 70 percent of your body weight on the left leg and 30 percent on the right.

6

7 For the transition into Parting Mustang's Mane (Right), shift your body weight back onto the right leg, with your left heel touching the ground.

8 Turn your left foot inward 85 degrees to the right, then shift your body weight back onto your left leg (see figure *a*). Turn your upper body also to the right and raise your right foot slightly. Turn it to the right so that it is about perpendicular to your upper body, and then move it back toward your left leg and end with your right toes touching the ground. Turn your left hand over simultaneously so that your left palm faces the ground and your right palm faces your left palm, as if holding a large ball on the left side of your body (see figure *b*).

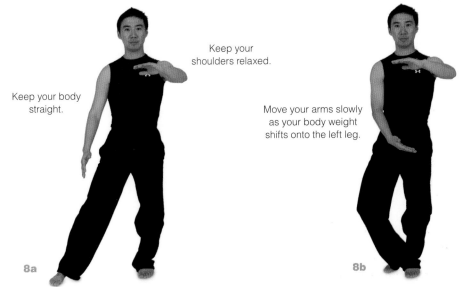

Keep your body straight.

Keep your shoulders relaxed.

Move your arms slowly as your body weight shifts onto the left leg.

8a

8b

9 For completion of Parting Mustang's Mane (Right), take a full step with your right leg to the right side, touching the ground with your heel first (see figure *a*). Move your body weight gradually onto your right foot, move your right arm up and left arm down, and end the movement with your right hand in front of your body and your left hand alongside your left hip (see figure *b*). End with about 70 percent of your body weight on the right leg and 30 percent on the left.

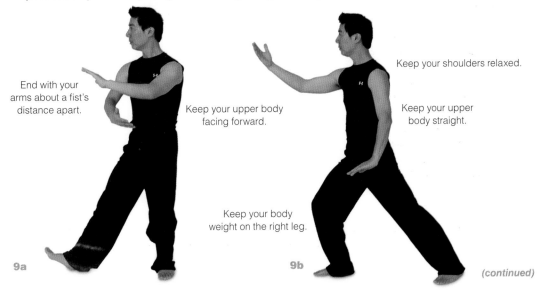

End with your arms about a fist's distance apart.

Keep your upper body facing forward.

Keep your shoulders relaxed.

Keep your upper body straight.

Keep your body weight on the right leg.

9a

9b

(continued)

10 Repeat steps 2 through 9 several times. Steps 2 through 6 are *Ye Ma Fen Zong* (Left) and steps 7 through 9 are *Ye Ma Fen Zong* (Right).

11 To end the form, continue from step 9 and move your body weight back equally onto your left leg; turn your upper body left 90 degrees so you are facing forward; move your left arm up and turn your right one inward to end with both arms at shoulder level, palms facing the ground (see figure *a*); turn your right foot inward to be perpendicular with your upper body and bring it in a half step toward your left leg; distribute your body weight equally onto your legs; unbend your knees; and move your arms down to the relaxed hanging starting position (see figure *b*). Breathe naturally, and breathe out when the arms move down.

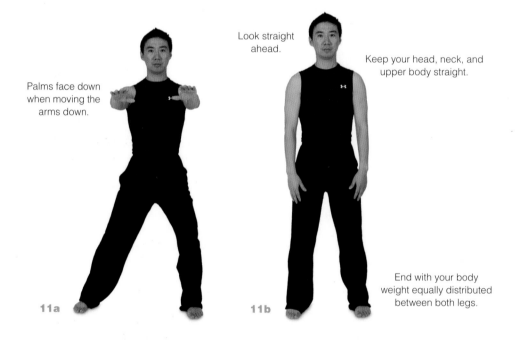

Palms face down when moving the arms down.

Look straight ahead.

Keep your head, neck, and upper body straight.

11a

11b

End with your body weight equally distributed between both legs.

Brush Knee and Twist Step

Lou Qi You Bu

The name of this form comes from its key movement characteristics: moving one hand in a circle in front of the knees while taking twist steps. The movement itself is rooted in the martial arts background of tai chi. Imagine your opponent is attacking you with his right leg or fist; you then protect yourself using your left hand. Rather than directly fighting back using your left hand, you move your opponent's leg or fist to the side and then you bring back your left hand via a circular movement so that your left hand will not be hurt. This move also exposes your opponent's head or chest. The completed movement to this point is called *Lou Qii* or *Brush Knee*. You then fight back by moving your left leg a half step forward and moving your right hand forward toward the area exposed by the first part of this movement. This move ends in a left bow foot, which you learned in chapter 3. In Chinese martial arts, when a stance has the opposite hand and leg in the front (left leg and right hand in this example), it is known as a twist step. This is why the second movement of this form is called *Twist Step*.

TIP Keep your shoulders relaxed and at the same level, and hold your upper body tall and straight so that you can practice the form in a relaxed way.

1 **For the starting position, stand with your legs shoulder-width apart and feet parallel to each other. Keep your upper body, head, and neck upright. Hold your chin slightly down and relax your face with a slight smile. Hang your arms down along your sides with your hands resting naturally beside your thighs. Keep your body weight equally distributed between both legs. Clear your mind and keep a peaceful mental state throughout the whole form.**

Breathe naturally.

Keep your head straight and hold your chin low.

Keep your shoulders relaxed.

(continued)

2 Raise your arms slowly in front of your body until they are level with your shoulders; your arms will be parallel to each other, shoulder-width apart, and your palms will be facing down. Keep your upper body, head, and neck upright. Hold your chin slightly down and relax your face with a slight smile. Keep your body weight distributed equally between both legs.

Breathe in while your arms move up.

Do not bend your wrists.

Keep your head held high, facing forward, and chin held slightly down.

2

3 Slowly squat while you move both arms down simultaneously to waist level. Keep your upper body upright while squatting. Your body weight is equally distributed on both legs.

Keep your head straight.

Keep your upper body straight.

Do not squat so far that your knees go past your toes.

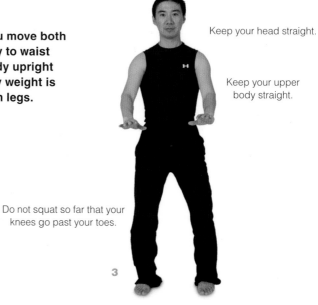

3

4 For the Brush Knee and Twist Step (Left), move your body weight onto your right leg; turn your upper body 90 degrees to the right; turn your left hand up, move your left arm up, and then turn your left hand down while turning your right hand up and moving your right arm down then up (see figure *a*); and take a half step back with your left leg, ending with your left toes touching the ground while your eyes are looking at your right hand (see figure *b*).

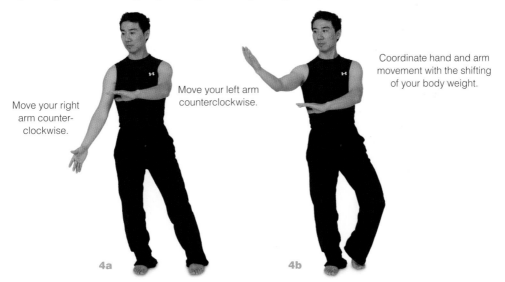

Move your right arm counter-clockwise.

Move your left arm counterclockwise.

Coordinate hand and arm movement with the shifting of your body weight.

4a

4b

5 Take a full step to the left with your left leg, heel touching the ground first then placing your whole foot down (see figure *a*); turn your upper body to the left and push your right hand out straight at ear level (see figure *b*); move your left hand over your left knee; and end the movement with your legs in a left bow step (see figure *c*), with your right arm reaching straight out, palm facing out, and your left hand facing the ground at waist level on your left side.

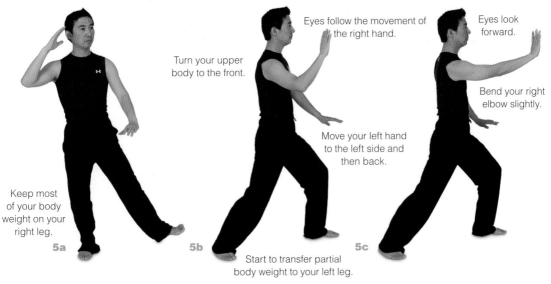

Keep most of your body weight on your right leg.

Turn your upper body to the front.

Eyes follow the movement of the right hand.

Move your left hand to the left side and then back.

Eyes look forward.

Bend your right elbow slightly.

5a

5b

Start to transfer partial body weight to your left leg.

5c

(continued)

6 For the transition into the Brush Knee and Twist Step (Right), move your body weight back onto your right leg with your left heel touching the ground (see figure a), turn your left foot right about 45 degrees, turn your upper body about 180 degrees while transferring body weight back onto your left leg, and take a half step toward your left leg with your right leg, with your right toe touching the ground (see figure b). Meanwhile, move your right arm down along a clockwise arc and your left arm over and moving up along a counterclockwise path.

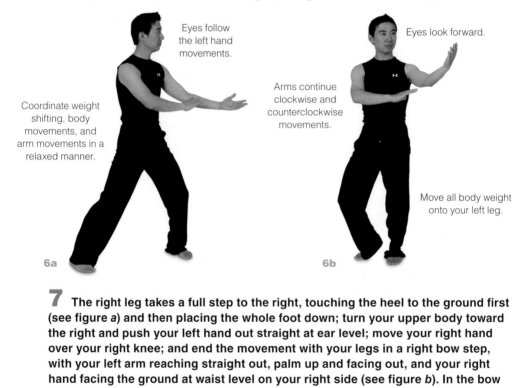

Eyes follow the left hand movements.

Coordinate weight shifting, body movements, and arm movements in a relaxed manner.

Eyes look forward.

Arms continue clockwise and counterclockwise movements.

Move all body weight onto your left leg.

6a

6b

7 The right leg takes a full step to the right, touching the heel to the ground first (see figure a) and then placing the whole foot down; turn your upper body toward the right and push your left hand out straight at ear level; move your right hand over your right knee; and end the movement with your legs in a right bow step, with your left arm reaching straight out, palm up and facing out, and your right hand facing the ground at waist level on your right side (see figure b). In the bow

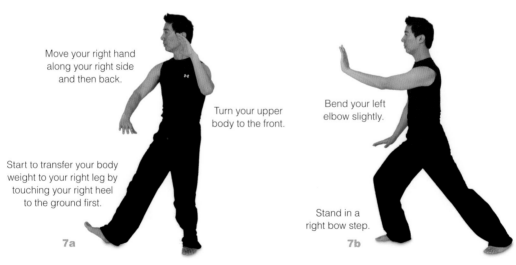

Move your right hand along your right side and then back.

Turn your upper body to the front.

Start to transfer your body weight to your right leg by touching your right heel to the ground first.

Bend your left elbow slightly.

Stand in a right bow step.

7a

7b

step, left and right hand movements are executed simultaneously. When doing the bow step, the face, front foot, and pushed-out hand move in the same direction. Make sure there is about the distance of a full step between the feet when in a bow step.

8 Repeat steps 2 through 5 several times. Steps 2 through 3 are for *Lou Qi You Bu* (Left) and steps 4 through 5 are for *Lou Qi You Bu* (Right).

9 To end the form, continue from step 6 and move your body weight back equally onto your legs; turn your upper body left 90 degrees to face forward; move your left arm up and turn your right arm inward to end with both arms at shoulder level, palms facing the ground (see figure *a*); turn your right foot inward to be perpendicular to your upper body and bring it in a half step toward your left leg; distribute your body weight equally between both legs; unbend your knees; and move your arms down to the relaxed hanging starting position (see figure *b*). Breathe naturally, and breathe out when the arms move down.

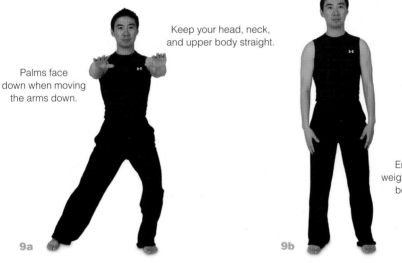

Keep your head, neck, and upper body straight.

Palms face down when moving the arms down.

End with your body weight equally distributed between both legs.

9a

9b

Reverse Reeling Forearm in Place

Dao Juan Gong

The name of this form reflects the movement of both the legs and the arms. *Dao* in Chinese means "moving back," *Gong* is "arm," and *Juan* means "curving." Together, *Juan Gong* means "curved arms." It is said that tai chi masters discovered this movement from watching monkeys play fighting: One monkey moves back or withdraws as a trick to entice the other monkey into moving forward. As the advancing monkey feels that she is winning the play fight, she relaxes and becomes comfortable, and that is when the retreating monkey fights back. Therefore, another name for this form is *Do Lian Hou* (Drive Monkeys Away), referring to fending monkeys off with one hand while at the same time enticing the monkeys to come closer with the other hand.

The movements of this form are a combination of the backward footwork you learned in chapter 3 and Back-and-Forth Vertical Side Ellipse Movement in Sequence in chapter 4. To facilitate learning, however, you will learn this form while standing in place, so instead of moving your legs backward, you will only need to shift your body weight from one leg to another. In chapters 10 and 11, which integrate several previously learned forms, you will learn the movements of the original form.

TIP Coordinate hand and arm movements with turning of the body. Arms move along curved paths so that as one moves forward, the other moves backward, which defines the retreating yet beckoning aspect of this form.

1 **For the starting position, stand with your legs shoulder-width apart and your feet parallel to each other. Keep your upper body, head, and neck straight. Hold your chin slightly down and relax your face with a slight smile. Hang your arms down along your sides with your hands resting naturally beside your thighs. Keep your body weight equally distributed between both legs. Clear your mind and keep a peaceful mental state throughout the whole form.**

Keep your shoulders relaxed.

Breathe naturally.

Keep your head straight and chin low.

1

2 Raise your arms slowly in front of your body until they are level with your shoulders; your arms will be parallel to each other, shoulder-width apart, and your palms will be facing down. Keep your upper body, head, and neck straight. Hold your chin slightly down and relax your face with a slight smile. Keep your body weight distributed equally between both legs.

Keep your head held high, facing forward, and chin held slightly down.

Breathe in while your arms move up.

Do not bend your wrists.

2

Keep your head straight.

Do not squat so far that your knees go past your toes.

3

3 Squat down slowly while moving both arms down simultaneously to the level of your waist. Keep your upper body upright while squatting.

4 Turn both hands over so that your palms face up; draw your right hand back slowly toward your waist (see figure *a*), then back up slightly over your right shoulder; at the same time, turn your upper body right 90 degrees, shifting your body weight onto your right leg; move your left leg a half step toward your right leg, touching the ground with your left toes; and look into your right palm with your eyes (see figure *b*).

Move your right hand along an arc, down first and then up.

Keep your upper body upright and shoulders relaxed.

Shift body weight onto your right leg.

4a

4b

(continued)

5 Repeat step 3 for the left side by moving your right hand up (see figure *a*) and then pushing it forward when your right hand is above your right ear. Meanwhile, draw your left hand back, move it slowly down to your waist, and then bring it back up slightly over your left shoulder; at the same time, turn your upper body left 90 degrees and shift your body weight onto your left leg (see figure *b*). When complete, your right toes should be touching the ground. Your eyes should look into your left palm. Hands should be vertical at the end of the forward push, with all fingers extended yet relaxed (see figure *c*).

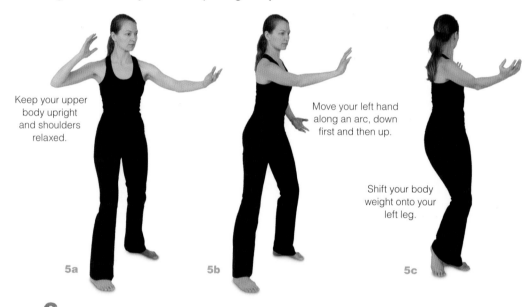

Keep your upper body upright and shoulders relaxed.

Move your left hand along an arc, down first and then up.

Shift your body weight onto your left leg.

5a   5b   5c

6 Start to move your left hand forward (see figure *a*) and push it forward as soon as your left hand passes your ear (see figure *b*); meanwhile, move your right hand back slowly to your waist. Return your right leg to the starting position (see figure *c*).

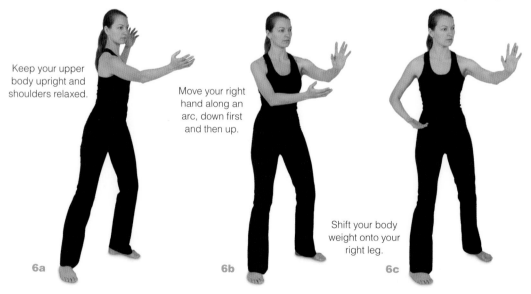

Keep your upper body upright and shoulders relaxed.

Move your right hand along an arc, down first and then up.

Shift your body weight onto your right leg.

6a   6b   6c

7 Both arms are stretched out forward at shoulder level (see figure *a*); move them down into the starting position (see figure *b*).

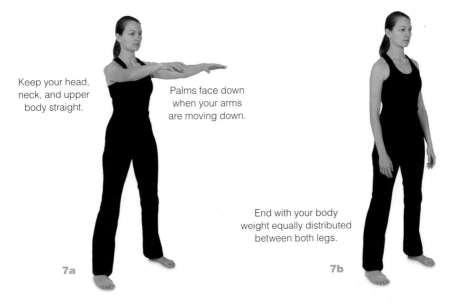

Keep your head, neck, and upper body straight.

Palms face down when your arms are moving down.

End with your body weight equally distributed between both legs.

7a

7b

8 Repeat steps 1 through 6 several times.

Parting Mustang's Mane (page 84)

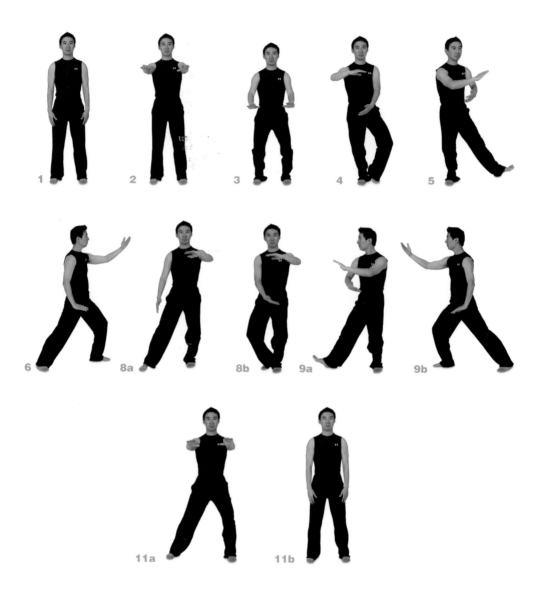

Brush Knee and Twist Step (page 89)

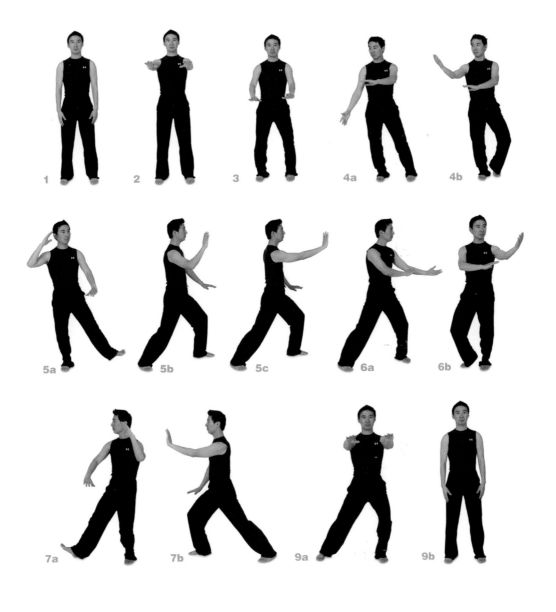

Reverse Reeling Forearm in Place (page 94)

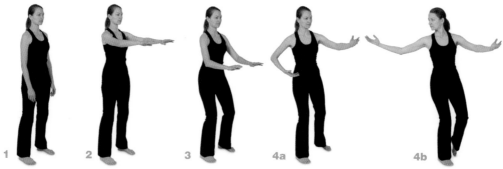

1   2   3   4a   4b

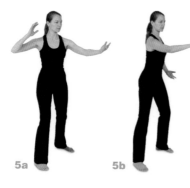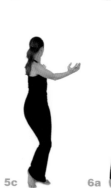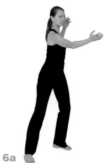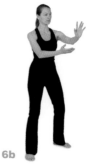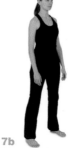

5a   5b   5c   6a   6b

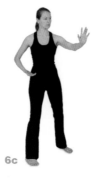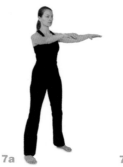

6c   7a   7b

chapter 7

Forms for Stress Relief and Low-Back Health

In this chapter, you will learn three popular tai chi forms. This set of forms is characterized by movements coordinating the hands, arms, and legs with waist twisting and weight shifting. These movements actively involve the low back. More important, many of these movements are believed to stimulate the flow of qi along the Liver meridian. TCM believes that the liver is directly related to temperament and stress level. By regularly promoting qi circulation along the Liver meridian, your stress level should be controllable.

Due to our modern sedentary lifestyle, low-back pain has become one of the most common medical complaints, affecting 70 to 85 percent of all people at some point during their lives. Low-back pain is the fifth most common reason for all physician visits in the United States, and approximately one-quarter of U.S. adults reported experiencing low-back pain lasting at least one whole day in the past three months. Low-back pain is also costly: In 2005, Americans spent $85.9 billion looking for relief from back and neck pain through surgery, doctor's visits, X-rays, MRI scans, and medications, up from $52.1 billion in 1997, according to a study by Martin et al. published in the *Journal of the American Medical Association* (JAMA) in 2008. That money hasn't helped reduce the number of sufferers, however; in 2005, 15 percent of U.S. adults reported back problems—up from 12 percent in 1997. Low-back pain can also limit physical activity, and it is the most frequent cause of activity limitation in people under the age of 45.

Stress, another side effect of modern society, is the emotional and physical strain caused by our response to pressure from the outside world. Common stress reactions include tension, irritability, inability to concentrate, and a variety of physical symptoms such as headaches and a rapid heartbeat. Life is full of stress, and it is usually unavoidable. In fact, short bouts of low-level stress are normal and could be good for health. You may have heard the phrase *fight or flight* before; it is a common response to danger. When you are afraid that someone or something may physically hurt you, your body naturally responds with a burst of energy so that you will be better able to survive the dangerous situation (fight) or escape from it (flight). When dealing with stress, the body reacts by releasing chemicals into the blood. These chemicals provide more energy and strength, which can be a good thing if stress is caused by physical danger.

However, if stress gets out of control, you may have too many of these chemicals in your body, which can harm your health. Studies have found that long-term stressful situations can produce a lasting, low-level stress that is hard on the body. The nervous system senses continued stress and remains slightly activated, continuing to pump out extra stress hormones over an extended time. This can wear out the body's reserves, leaving a person feeling depleted or overwhelmed; weaken the immune system; and cause other problems, which can be expressed in both mental symptoms (e.g., tension, irritability, excessive tiredness, trouble sleeping) and physical symptoms (e.g., pounding heart, difficulty breathing, upset stomach, tight muscles causing pain and trembling). According to studies, such as the stress surveys conducted by American Psychological Association (2012), millions of Americans suffer from stress each year, and three out of four adults said they experienced stress at least twice a month. Some studies have reported that the number of people in the United States reporting that stress affects their work has gone up more than four times over the past two decades.

Fortunately, studies have shown that regular physical activity can help reduce low-back pain and stress. There is strong evidence that leisure-time physical activity has a primary preventive effect on low-back pain. For those who suffer from low-back pain, a number of recent studies show that a lack of core strength contributes to pain and stiffness in the low back. Therefore, a possible long-term solution for back pain lies in strengthening and stretching exercises for the abdominal muscles, hips, and low back. Some pains or aches in your low back might be the result of weak abdominal muscles. When you have weak abdominal muscles, you are more likely to have poor posture and your back muscles are forced to take over, which can strain them in a way that becomes uncomfortable or painful over time. You can minimize back pain by doing exercises that make your abs stronger while also training to increase the strength and flexibility of your low back, hips, and thighs. Everyone's back pain is different, so it is a good idea to check with your health care provider about what is best for you before starting a low-back exercise program.

Studies also have shown that there are some direct stress-relief benefits to exercise. There are a number of reasons for this, according to a Mayo Clinic summary (Mayo Clinic). First, exercise increases the production of the brain's feel-good neurotransmitters, called *endorphins*. Although this production is often referred to as a *runner's high*, any physical activity can produce this feeling. Second, exercise creates meditation through motion. As you begin to shed your daily tensions through regular movement and physical activity, you may find that this focus on a single task and the resulting energy from it may help you be calm and clear in everything that you do. Finally, regular exercise can increase self-confidence and lower the symptoms associated with mild depression and anxiety. Exercise also can improve your sleep, which is often disrupted by stress, depression, and anxiety. Regular exercise can give you a sense of command over your body and your life.

What about tai chi, then? Because tai chi is a moderate exercise involving all major muscle groups in the body, it provides the same positive effects as many other exercises. Furthermore, tai chi is an exercise that pays a great deal of attention to waist movements, making it a means to improve low-back health. In fact, one of the forms introduced in this chapter, Deflect, Parry, and Punch, has been regularly used in China to treat low-back pain. As a mind–body exercise, tai chi can generate a motion medication effect. As soon as you learn and start to do the forms and routines, you will find yourself relaxing and enjoying the movement. There is also a strong theoretical foundation for these mental health benefits. According to TCM, the liver is directly related to the regulation of emotions. If a person gets angry or mad regularly, it will likely hurt the liver. Any exercise that helps the qi flow along the Liver meridian will likely help one's emotional well-being in dealing with stress. All three forms introduced in this chapter promote the flow of qi along the Liver meridian. Therefore, regular practice of these forms should help reduce stress.

Practice tai chi to make your low back healthier and reduce your stress!

Level

▶ Beginner

Benefits

▶ Strengthens the legs.

▶ Strengthens the arms.

▶ Improves balance.

▶ Improves body awareness.

▶ Reduces stress.

▶ Improves qi flow.

Contraindications

▶ Falling with loss of balance

Roll Back and Press

Lu Ji Shi

This form is named for two key movements: rolling back and pressing. Both movements stem from the martial arts origin of tai chi. They are based on the tai chi principle that you never fight back directly when your opponent is hitting you, and you do not simply avoid being hit since another hit likely will follow. Instead, you try to use your opponent's own strength against her and guide her into moving in a direction that allows you to easily fight back. *Lu* is a movement specifically designed for this purpose: You reach out to gauge the direction and strength of your opponent's attack and then guide it in a different direction. You may have experienced pushing a big ball down into water; you have to push on the middle of the ball, using all of your strength to push it into the water. If your strength is on one side of the ball, the ball escapes from your push by rolling away to the other side. *Lu* leads your opponent to one side of your body, either passing your side so that you can use your elbow or hands to fight back or moving back so that you can then fight back using *ji*, or pressing, which is the next movement in the form. When pressing, make sure both of your hands hit the middle of your opponent with your feet firmly planted so that your body weight becomes part of your fighting force. Together with the force of your opponent moving back, you should be able to fight back effectively and with power. Finally, *shi* simply means *forms* in Chinese.

TIP To perform Roll Back and Press correctly, the hands should move along horizontal circles in a natural, coordinated manner; the top hand moves along a larger circle while the lower one moves along a smaller circle. Rolling back, which is similar to falling back slightly, moves along a curve; the movement coordinates with the shifting of body weight.

1 For the starting position, stand with your legs shoulder-width apart and with your feet parallel to each other. Keep your upper body, head, and neck straight. Hold your chin slightly down and relax your face with a slight smile. Hang your arms down along your sides with your hands resting naturally beside your thighs. Keep your body weight equally distributed between both legs. Clear your mind and keep a peaceful mental state throughout the whole form.

2 Raise your arms slowly in front of your body until they are level with your shoulders; your arms will be parallel to each other, shoulder-width apart, and your palms will be facing down. Keep your upper body, head, and neck straight. Hold your chin slightly down and relax your face with a slight smile. Keep your body weight distributed equally between both legs.

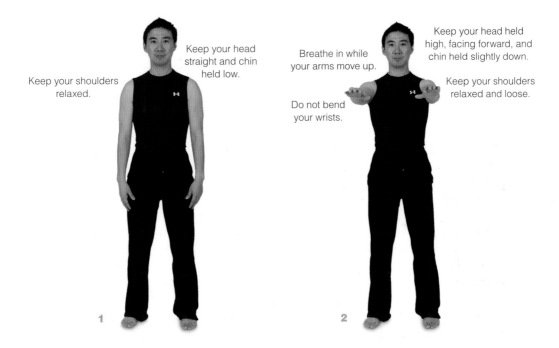

Keep your head straight and chin held low.

Keep your shoulders relaxed.

Breathe in while your arms move up.

Do not bend your wrists.

Keep your head held high, facing forward, and chin held slightly down.

Keep your shoulders relaxed and loose.

3 Slowly squat while you move both arms down simultaneously to waist level. Keep your upper body upright while squatting. Your body weight is equally distributed on both legs.

4 For the Roll Back and Press (Right), turn your left palm up, with your hand parallel to the ground; circle both arms clockwise parallel to the ground in front of you with your right arm on top; turn your upper body about 90 degrees to your right; and shift your body weight onto your left leg as you turn.

(continued)

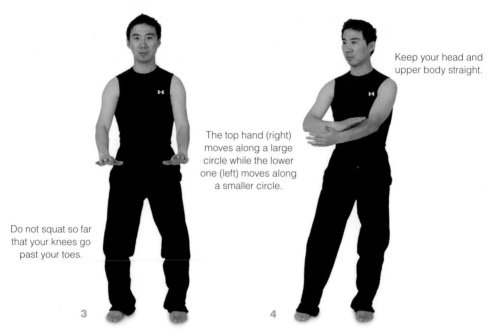

Keep your head and upper body straight.

The top hand (right) moves along a large circle while the lower one (left) moves along a smaller circle.

Do not squat so far that your knees go past your toes.

3

4

5 Keeping the majority of body weight on your left leg, move your hands so that your right hand and arm are in front of your right shoulder and your left hand is in front of your stomach.

6 For rolling back, roll both arms back while shifting your body weight entirely onto your left leg; end with only the toes of your right foot touching the ground.

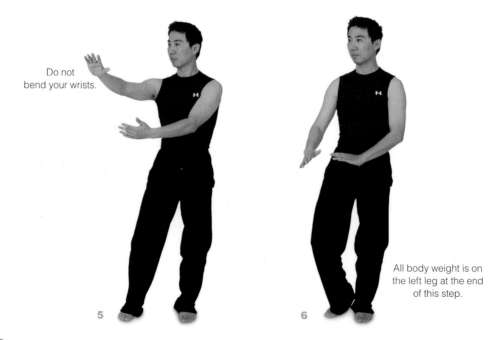

Do not bend your wrists.

All body weight is on the left leg at the end of this step.

5

6

7 For the press part of the movement, take a half step to the right with the right foot (see figure *a*), press both hands forward with palms facing each other, and end in a bow step with your right leg in front and both feet firmly placed on the ground. When your hands are pushed forward, they should synchronize with the shifting of your body weight; stop pushing your hands out when the bow step is complete (see figure *b*).

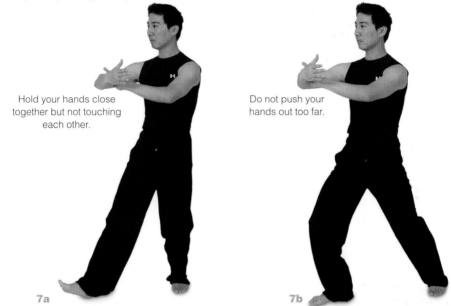

Hold your hands close together but not touching each other.

Do not push your hands out too far.

7a

7b

8 For the transition into the Roll Back and Press (Left), move your body weight onto your left leg; turn your right foot about 90 degrees to the front (see figure *a*); start to move your body weight back onto your right leg; turn your body 180

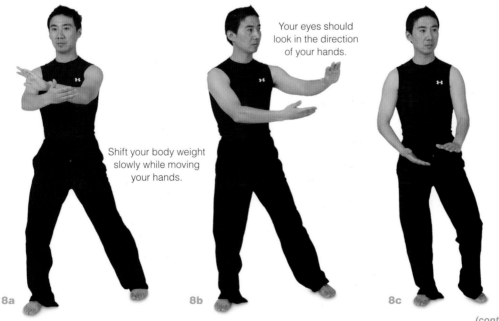

Your eyes should look in the direction of your hands.

Shift your body weight slowly while moving your hands.

8a

8b

8c

(continued)

degrees to the left; separate your hands; move them back, this time along a counterclockwise circular path with the left hand on top, left palm facing the ground, and right hand below, right palm facing up (see figures *b* and *c*); move your left hand to stop in front of your left shoulder and your right hand in front of your stomach; and roll both hands back along a clockwise path while shifting your body weight completely onto your right leg, with only the toes of your left foot touching the ground.

9 For the press, take a half step to the left with your left foot (see figure *a*), and press both hands forward with palms facing each other (see figure *b*).

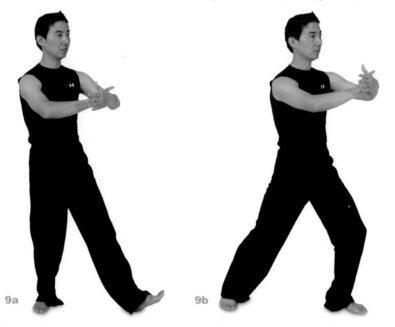

9a   9b

10 Repeat steps 3 through 8 several times, and when you're ready to complete the movement, move on to step 11.

11 For the closing position, move your body weight back onto your right leg, turn your upper body right 90 degrees to face forward, move both arms out at shoulder level with palms facing down (see figure *a*), turn your left foot 90 degrees toward the front, distribute your body weight equally between both legs, straighten your knees, and move your arms down, returning them to their starting position (see figure *b*).

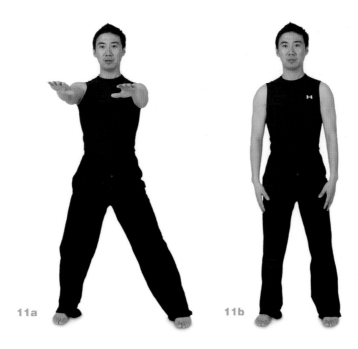

11a   11b

Grasp Sparrow's Tail

Lan Que Wei

The name of this form is an attempt to explain the movement using a fanciful example from real life. The movement itself, however, is closely associated with the martial arts origin of tai chi. Imagine that an opponent's attacking arm is a sparrow's tail and your hands are ropes. Through back-and-forth movements, you are trying to grasp the tail by pulling it (i.e., your opponent's arms) to control the opponent's body. Your legs do not make many changes during these movements; rather, a variety of hand and arm movements are employed in this form. However, when there is leg movement, make sure the hand movements coordinate with it (for example, pulling back the hands at the same time you bend the knee into a bow step).

TIP To keep your balance when performing Grasp Sparrow's Tail, there should be at least a foot (30 cm) between the parallel lines that the legs are standing on. Fully complete one movement before moving into the next one; distinguish movements clearly from each other, especially the hands and arms.

(continued)

Grasp Sparrow's Tail *(continued)*

1 For the starting position, stand with your legs shoulder-width apart and your feet parallel to each other. Keep your upper body, head, and neck straight. Hold your chin slightly down and relax your face with a slight smile. Hang your arms down along your sides with your hands resting naturally beside your thighs. Keep your body weight equally distributed between both legs. Clear your mind and keep a peaceful mental state throughout the whole form.

2 Raise your arms slowly in front of your body until they are level with your shoulders; your arms will be parallel to each other, shoulder-width apart, and your palms will be facing down. Keep your upper body, head, and neck straight. Hold your chin slightly down and relax your face with a slight smile. Keep your body weight distributed equally between both legs.

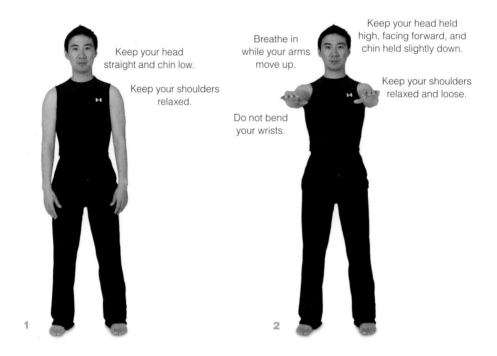

Keep your head straight and chin low.

Keep your shoulders relaxed.

Breathe in while your arms move up.

Keep your head held high, facing forward, and chin held slightly down.

Keep your shoulders relaxed and loose.

Do not bend your wrists.

3 Slowly squat while you move both arms down simultaneously to waist level. Keep your upper body upright while squatting. Your body weight is equally distributed on both legs.

4 For Grasp Sparrow's Tail (Right), shift your weight almost entirely onto your left leg while raising your right leg slightly with knee bent, and bring your leg in close to your left leg, putting only your right toes on the ground. Meanwhile, move your right hand down and your left hand up into the familiar holding-ball position in front of the left side of your body.

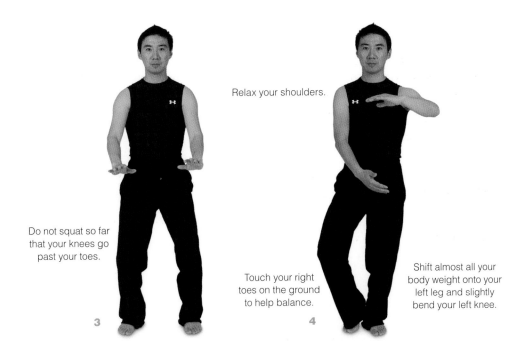

Relax your shoulders.

Do not squat so far that your knees go past your toes.

Touch your right toes on the ground to help balance.

Shift almost all your body weight onto your left leg and slightly bend your left knee.

3

4

5 With your arms crossed in front of your body, take a full step to the right with the right leg so that your heel touches the ground first (see figure *a*) and shift your body weight gradually onto your right leg, ending in a right bow step. Meanwhile, push your right arm up and forward along a curve and press your left hand down (see figure *b*). This style of the move is called *bing* in tai chi.

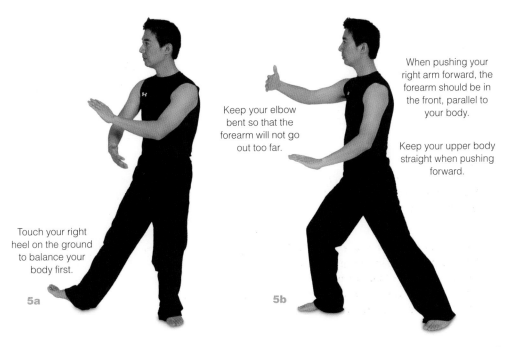

Keep your elbow bent so that the forearm will not go out too far.

When pushing your right arm forward, the forearm should be in the front, parallel to your body.

Keep your upper body straight when pushing forward.

Touch your right heel on the ground to balance your body first.

5a

5b

(continued)

6 To pull back, turn both palms so that they are facing each other (see figure *a*) and pull both hands back and down together to your left front side while shifting your body weight back onto your left leg (see figure *b*).

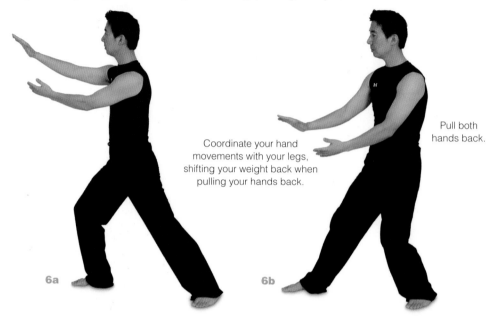

Coordinate your hand movements with your legs, shifting your weight back when pulling your hands back.

Pull both hands back.

6a

6b

7 To press forward, turn your right palm toward yourself and your left palm away (see figure *a*). With your palms touching, push your right hand forward using your left hand while shifting your body weight onto your right leg, ending in a right bow step (see figure *b*).

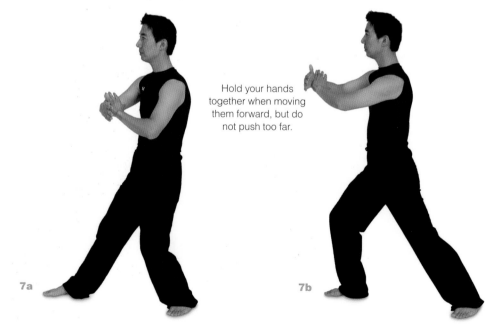

Hold your hands together when moving them forward, but do not push too far.

7a

7b

8 To pull back, release both hands by pushing them forward with palms facing the ground (see figure *a*); shift your body weight back onto your left leg and raise your right toes, with only your right heel touching the ground, while pulling both hands back into your body (see figure *b*).

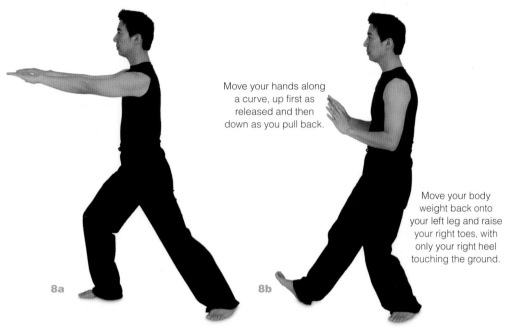

Move your hands along a curve, up first as released and then down as you pull back.

Move your body weight back onto your left leg and raise your right toes, with only your right heel touching the ground.

8a

8b

9 To push forward, push both hands down (called *an* in tai chi), shift your body weight onto your right leg (see figure *a*), and end in a right bow step with both hands up, palms pushing outward (see figure *b*). When pushing forward using your forearms, your strength should be in your arms; when pushing forward using your palms, the strength should be in the bottom of the palm. Make sure all pushing movements follow curved paths.

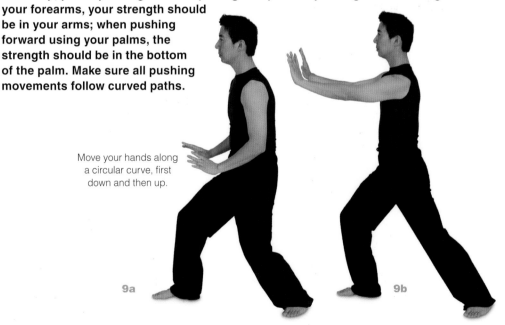

Move your hands along a circular curve, first down and then up.

9a

9b

(continued)

Grasp Sparrow's Tail *(continued)*

10 For the transition, move your body weight back to your left leg, turn your right foot to the left about 90 degrees, and turn your upper body and arms left to face the front.

11 Repeat steps 3 through 9 for the other side of your body for Grasp Sparrow's Tail (Left), starting from shifting your body weight onto your right leg, touching your left toes to the ground, and holding a ball, so to speak, on the right side of your body.

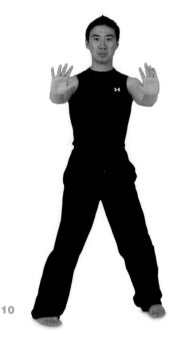

10

12 For the closing position, move your body weight back onto your right leg, turn your upper body right 90 degrees to face forward, move both arms out at shoulder level with palms facing down (see figure *a*), turn your left foot 90 degrees toward the front, distribute your body weight equally between your legs, straighten your knees, and move your arms down to return them to their starting position (see figure *b*).

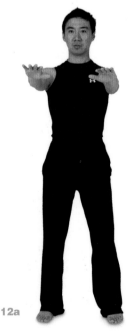

12a

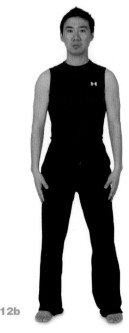

12b

Deflect, Parry, and Punch

Ban Lan Chui

The name of this form comes directly from its original martial arts meaning. *Ban* means "deflecting," *lan* refers to parrying the opponents' attack, and *chui* refers to punching opponents. Note that their exact meanings and applications in tai chi are slightly different from the ones in other martial arts applications. Instead of deflecting and parrying using maximal strength, tai chi deflecting and parrying movements always try to use the opponents' strength against them and guide the coming attack in a direction that allows you to fight back using minimal effort. A well-known Chinese saying is, "With the right skill, a light thing can move a heavy thing," which derives from this principle of minimal effort.

TIP To perform the Deflect, Parry, and Punch form correctly, coordinate arm movements with leg movements, especially when shifting body weight. Changing from one lead side to the other should be conducted in a natural, relaxed, and smooth manner. Keep movements soft and comfortable.

1 For the starting position, stand with your legs shoulder-width apart and your feet parallel to each other. Keep your upper body, head, and neck straight. Hold your chin slightly down and relax your face with a slight smile. Hang your arms down along your sides with your hands resting naturally beside your thighs. Keep your body weight equally distributed between both legs. Clear your mind and keep a peaceful mental state throughout the whole form.

Keep your head straight and chin held low.

Keep your shoulders relaxed.

(continued)

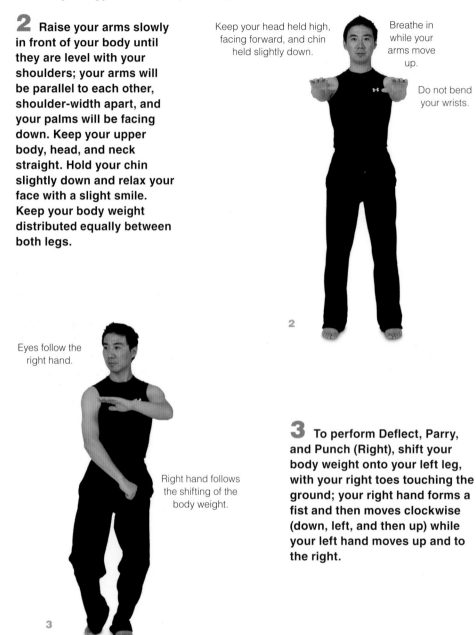

2 Raise your arms slowly in front of your body until they are level with your shoulders; your arms will be parallel to each other, shoulder-width apart, and your palms will be facing down. Keep your upper body, head, and neck straight. Hold your chin slightly down and relax your face with a slight smile. Keep your body weight distributed equally between both legs.

Keep your head held high, facing forward, and chin held slightly down.

Breathe in while your arms move up.

Do not bend your wrists.

Eyes follow the right hand.

Right hand follows the shifting of the body weight.

3 To perform Deflect, Parry, and Punch (Right), shift your body weight onto your left leg, with your right toes touching the ground; your right hand forms a fist and then moves clockwise (down, left, and then up) while your left hand moves up and to the right.

4 Move your arms arcing out and forward while taking a full step forward with your right leg, with right heel touching the ground first (see figure *a*); gradually move your body weight onto your right leg and end in a right bow step (see figure *b*); both hands follow the weight shift, ending with the right fist up and out and left hand close to the right elbow; and your eyes watch your right fist throughout the movement.

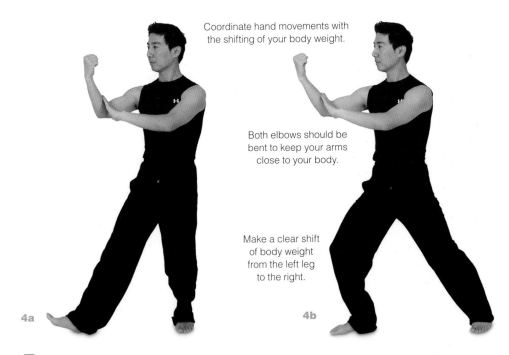

Coordinate hand movements with the shifting of your body weight.

Both elbows should be bent to keep your arms close to your body.

Make a clear shift of body weight from the left leg to the right.

4a

4b

5 To transition into Deflect, Parry, and Punch (Left), shift your body weight back onto your left leg, turn your right foot about 45 degrees to the left, and then move your body weight back onto your right leg so that now your left leg has only the left toes touching the ground (see figure *a*). Meanwhile, release your right fist and move both hands away from each other; your left hand becomes a fist and moves along a vertical circle in front of body from left to right (counterclockwise). (See figure *b*.)

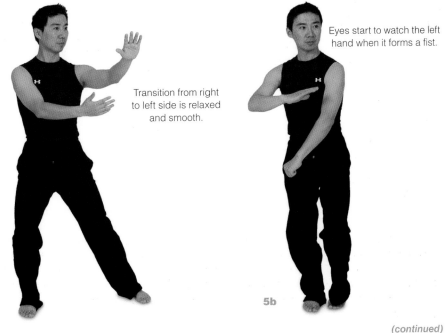

Transition from right to left side is relaxed and smooth.

Eyes start to watch the left hand when it forms a fist.

5a

5b

(continued)

6 To finish the movement, start by repeating step 3 but from the left side of your body. Move your arms while your left leg takes a full step forward; touch your left heel to the ground first (see figure *a*); gradually shift your body weight onto your left leg, put down your whole left foot, and end in a left bow step (see figure *b*); both hands follow the shift of body weight, ending with your left fist up and your right hand close to your left elbow; and your eyes are on your left fist.

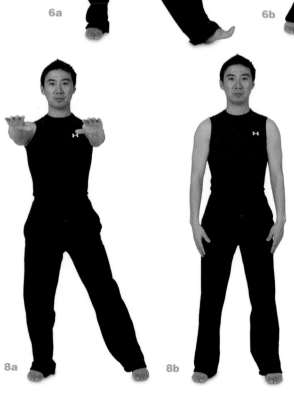

6a

6b

7 Repeat steps 3 through 6 for both sides several times.

8 For the closing position, move your body weight back onto your right leg, turn your upper body right 90 degrees to face forward, move both arms out at shoulder level with palms facing down (see figure *a*), turn your left foot 90 degrees toward the front and distribute your body weight equally between both legs, straighten your knees, and move your arms down, returning them to their starting position (see figure *b*).

8a

8b

Roll Back and Press (page 104)

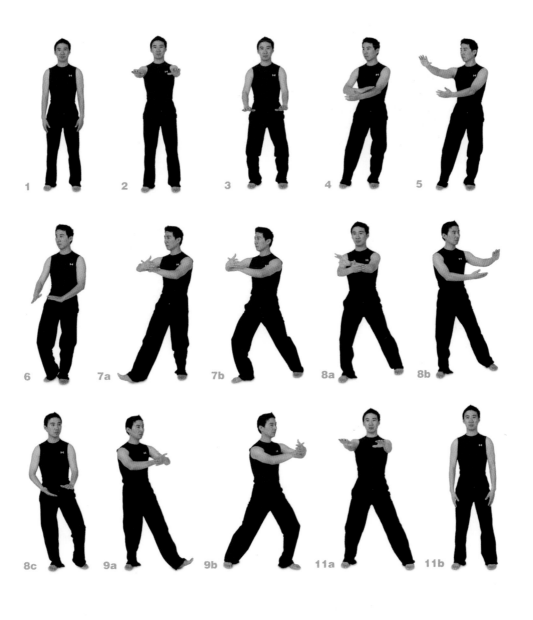

1

2

3

4

5

6

7a

7b

8a

8b

8c

9a

9b

11a

11b

Grasp Sparrow's Tail (page 109)

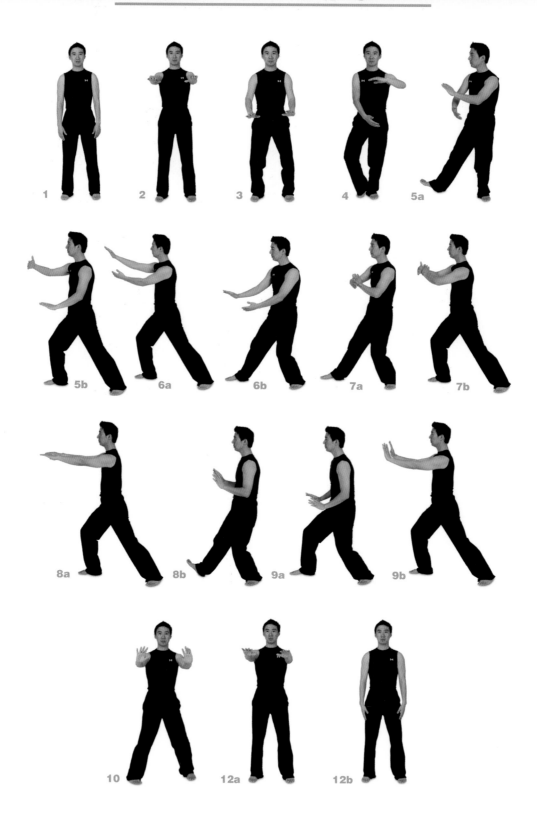

1 2 3 4 5a

5b 6a 6b 7a 7b

8a 8b 9a 9b

10 12a 12b

Deflect, Parry, and Punch (page 115)

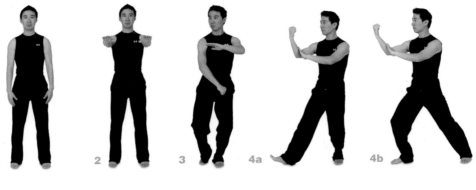

1   2   3   4a   4b

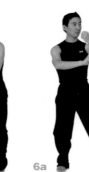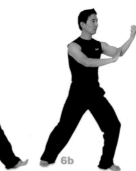

5a   5b   6a   6b

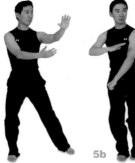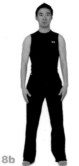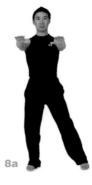

8a   8b

chapter 8

Forms for Balance

Interest in tai chi in the United States, as mentioned in chapter 1, arose after the widespread reporting of a study on the significant impact of tai chi on improving balance. Because of tai chi movement characteristics such as shifting body weight from one leg to another, any tai chi practice will help improve your balance. Instead of simply repeating the general balance-improvement movements presented so far in this book, this chapter introduces two forms that can help specifically improve balance.

Balance is the ability to maintain a posture without falling. When we are healthy and younger, we are able to maintain balance because the brain is continually receiving and processing signals from at least three major sources: the eyes, the muscles and joints, and the vestibular system (inner ear and brain). The brain then determines how the body needs to be positioned relative to the ground to maintain balance. Over time, many adults decrease their exercise and activity levels. This in turn diminishes their muscle strength, coordination, and joint flexibility. The vestibular, somatosensory, and visual systems decline with age, leading to a decrease in balance (Schmitz, 2007), and therefore we see more falls in older adults.

According to an article on the Centers for Disease Control website, approximately one-third of adults over the age of 65 fall each year, and many of those individuals fall more than once per year. Those are just the falls that are reported; actual falls are higher. Although everyone falls, the consequences of an unintentional fall in older adults tend to be more serious than in younger populations. For example, falls in older adults may lead to loss of independence, illness, and early death. Falls are the leading cause of both fatal and nonfatal injuries for people over the age of 65 and the number one reason older adults are admitted to nursing homes. Falls should not be seen as only a problem for older adults, however; fall prevention should start at earlier ages, such as 40 or 50.

Fortunately, falling risks can be significantly reduced by taking preventive measures, and regular exercise is one of the best measures. All exercise is helpful, but tai chi has proven to be one of the most effective forms of exercise for fall prevention. There are three possible reasons for this. First, during tai chi practice, body weight is constantly shifting from one leg to the other. As a result, all systems related to maintaining balance are constantly processing the ever-changing signals concerning body position relative to the ground. Second, in contrast to the one-dimensional movements commonly done in many other exercises (e.g., weightlifting), tai chi involves movement in all directions. As a result, small muscle groups around the joints are strengthened to a greater degree, which helps in maintaining and regaining balance in all directions. Third, hand and arm movements during tai chi practice are coordinated, which also helps maintain balance. Finally, bone health of older adults should benefit from tai chi because the chance of a fall-related bone injury (e.g., hip fractures) decreases along with the reduced risk of falling, because tai chi is an excellent weight-bearing exercise, and because older adults may increase their physical activity thanks to their reduced fear of falling, which has further positive impact on their bone health.

As mentioned previously, in this chapter, you will learn two tai chi forms designed specifically to improve balance. Start your practice by finding an open space of at least 1 square yard or meter that has firm ground. Practice can be done anywhere, inside or outside. It is okay to practice without shoes as long as the surface is safe for bare or stocking feet. If you are experiencing a balance problem now, you can start the practice by focusing on leg movement first while holding onto a chair in front of you or bracing yourself by placing a hand on a wall. You can gradually increase practice difficulty by lifting your legs higher and eventually closing your eyes. Apply the tai chi movements you have learned into your daily life. For example, you can perform Standing on One Leg while you are brushing your teeth and Kicking With Feet while you watch TV. Practice tai chi and improve your balance!

Standing on One Leg

Jin Ji Du Li

The Chinese name of this form, *Jin Ji Du Li*, derives from its posture. The direct translation of the name is, "A golden rooster stands on one foot." This is also a well-known posture in Chinese martial arts. Six major meridians pass through the legs, and it is believed that this form helps qi flow through these meridians. It's also a good form for someone who wants quick results—you should be able to feel the impact of this move in just a few seconds when you perform it with your eyes closed.

1 **Stand with your legs shoulder-width apart and feet parallel, with your body weight divided evenly between both legs. Keep your upper body, head, and neck straight. Hold your chin slightly down and relax your face with a slight smile. Hang your arms down along your sides with your hands resting naturally beside your thighs. Clear your mind and keep a peaceful mental state throughout the whole form. Breathe naturally and focus on your Dan Tian.**

Keep your shoulders relaxed and loose.

Keep your head held straight, facing forward, and chin held slightly down.

(continued)

2 Raise your arms slowly in front of your body until they are level with your shoulders; your arms will be parallel to each other, shoulder-width apart, and your palms will be facing down. Keep your upper body, head, and neck straight. Hold your chin slightly down and relax your face with a slight smile. Keep your body weight distributed equally between both legs. Breathe naturally, but breathe in when your arms move up.

3 For Standing on One Leg (Left), shift your body weight gradually onto your left leg. Slightly turn your upper body to the right, and lower your arms and hands to waist level, keeping palms parallel to the ground. Your right hand should be slightly in front of and above your right hip. Move your right hand, with the palm still facing the ground, in a slow clockwise circle. Move your head slightly downward so as to be able to watch the path your hand is making.

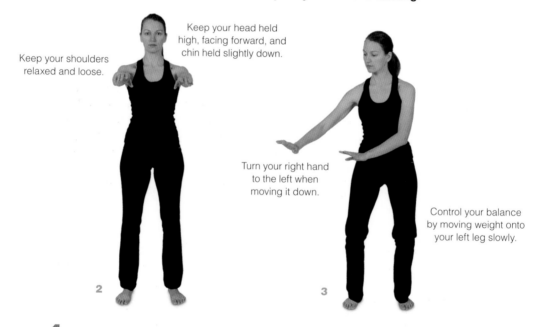

Keep your head held high, facing forward, and chin held slightly down.

Keep your shoulders relaxed and loose.

Turn your right hand to the left when moving it down.

Control your balance by moving weight onto your left leg slowly.

4 Move all of your body weight onto your left leg and slowly raise your right leg with your knee relaxed and bent. Raise your right hand at the same time at a slightly quicker speed than you are raising your right leg. Keep your left shoulder relaxed and slowly lower your left arm slightly, using this arm and hand to help keep your balance. Keep your left leg slightly bent also to help keep your balance. Practice this part with great caution since it is easy to lose your balance when standing on only one leg. You can start doing this part of the form while holding onto a chair in front of you or bracing yourself with your hand on a wall. Raise your right leg just 1 or 2 inches (3-5 cm) at first so you can quickly put it back down to regain your balance if needed. Repeat several times, gradually raising your leg higher and holding it up longer each time. Start to include the hand movements when you are comfortable and feel secure standing on one leg.

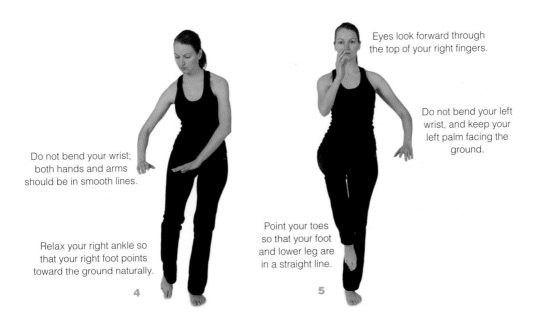

Do not bend your wrist; both hands and arms should be in smooth lines.

Relax your right ankle so that your right foot points toward the ground naturally.

4

Eyes look forward through the top of your right fingers.

Do not bend your left wrist, and keep your left palm facing the ground.

Point your toes so that your foot and lower leg are in a straight line.

5

5 Continue raising your right leg until your right thigh is parallel to the ground. Straighten your left leg so the knee is no longer bent. Keep raising your right arm, with it being naturally bent, at the same time you are raising your right leg until your fingertips are level with the tip of your nose. Move your left arm slightly down until your left hand is slightly in front of and over your left hip. Stand on only your left leg for up to 3 minutes (start with just a few seconds and increase the length as you improve), and then try closing your eyes for as long possible to increase the difficulty of the form.

6 To transition from left to right, place your right foot back on the ground lightly. Set your toes down first and then the rest of your right foot. Redistribute your body weight gradually onto your right leg. Move your right arm down slowly, with the palm of your right hand facing the ground, moving in sync with your leg as you lower it and put your right foot on the ground. Your eyes and head follow the movements of your right hand. Be aware of all the parts of your body involved in this transition and move them in a cohesive, smooth, coordinated manner.

Keep your body, neck, and head straight during the transition.

Keep your weight on your left leg until your right foot is fully grounded.

Touch your right toes to the ground first.

6

(continued)

7 For Standing on One Leg (Right), shift your body weight gradually onto your right leg. Slightly turn your upper body to the left. Your left hand should be slightly in front of and above your left hip. Move your left hand, with palm facing down and parallel to the ground, in a slow clockwise circle. Move your head slightly downward so as to be able to watch the path that your left hand is making.

8 Move all of your body weight onto your right leg. Raise your left leg slowly with your knee relaxed and bent. Raise your left hand at the same time at a slightly faster speed than you are raising your left leg. Keep your right shoulder relaxed and lower your right arms slightly and slowly. Use your right arm and hand to help keep your balance. Keep your right leg slightly bent to also help keep your balance. Practice this part with great caution since it is easy to lose your balance when standing on only one leg. You can start doing this part of the form while holding onto a chair in front of you or bracing yourself with your hand on a wall. Raise your left leg just 1 or 2 inches (3-5 cm) at first so you can quickly put it back down to regain your balance if needed. Raise your leg several times, gradually raising it higher and holding it up longer each time. Start to include the hand movements when you are comfortable and feel secure standing on one leg.

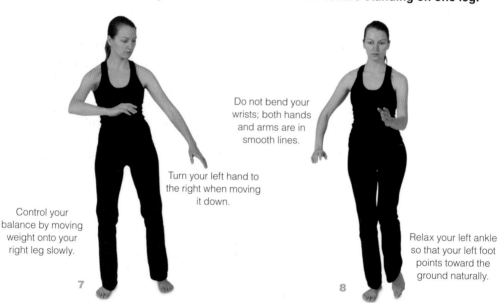

Do not bend your wrists; both hands and arms are in smooth lines.

Turn your left hand to the right when moving it down.

Control your balance by moving weight onto your right leg slowly.

Relax your left ankle so that your left foot points toward the ground naturally.

7

8

9 Continue raising your left leg until your left thigh is parallel to the ground. Straighten your right leg so the knee is no longer bent and keep it straight. Continue raising your left arm, keeping it naturally bent, at the same time you are raising your left leg until your fingertips are level with the tip of your nose. Move your right arm slightly down until your right hand is slightly in front of and over your right hip. Stand on only your right leg for up to 5 minutes (start for a few seconds and increase the length as you improve), then try closing your eyes for as long possible to increase the difficulty of the form.

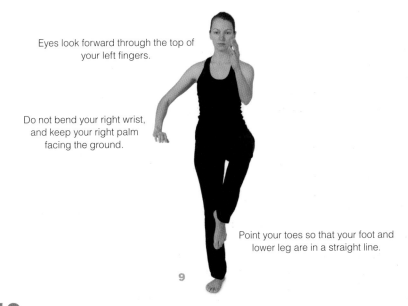

Eyes look forward through the top of your left fingers.

Do not bend your right wrist, and keep your right palm facing the ground.

Point your toes so that your foot and lower leg are in a straight line.

9

10 Practice Standing on One Leg several times, alternating the standing leg. Once you are ready to finish the movement, continue to step 11.

11 To close the form, place your left foot on the ground lightly, setting your toes down first and then the rest of the foot. Transfer your body weight gradually back onto your right leg, ending with your body weight equally distributed between both legs. Reach both arms out in front of your body at shoulder height, with palms facing the ground. Bring both hands and arms down alongside your body so that you are once again in the starting position for this form. Breathe naturally, but breathe out when you move your arms down. Hold the position for 1 to 2 minutes as you enjoy the peacefulness that comes through practice of this form.

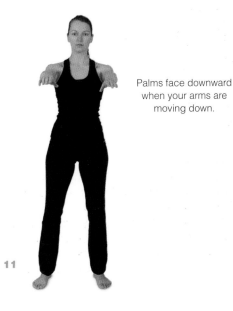

Palms face downward when your arms are moving down.

11

Kicking With Feet

Deng Jiao Li

The name of this form is Kicking With Feet; likely you can guess from the name how this form evolved from third-century martial arts practices and still is often used in modern martial arts. Nowadays, this form consists of movements that are slow, smooth, and fluid. Although no longer an effective means of self-defense, practicing this from every day will greatly improve your leg strength and balance, which will help protect you from falls. In China, practitioners of Chinese medicine often prescribe this exercise to patients who suffer from balance disorders or occasional dizziness.

TIP To achieve the best effect, keep the weight-bearing leg straight and firm, gripping the ground with your toes, and keep your upper body upright and straight. Avoid swaying as much as possible.

1 Stand with your legs shoulder-width apart and feet slightly turned out. Keep your upper body, head, and neck straight. Hold your chin slightly down and relax your face with a slight smile. Hang your hands naturally alongside your thighs with the palms facing inward. Keep your body weight balanced on both legs. Clear your mind and keep a peaceful mental state throughout the whole form. Breathe naturally and focus on your Dan Tian.

2 Raise your arms slowly in front of your body until they are level with your shoulders and both arms are parallel with palms facing the ground. Keep your upper body, head, and neck straight. Hold your chin slightly down and relax your

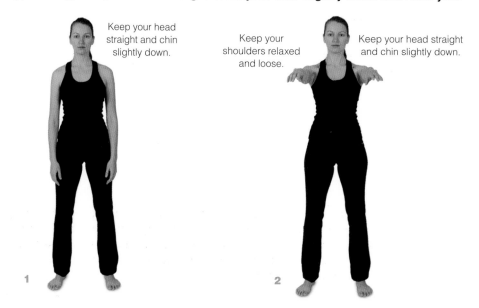

Keep your head straight and chin slightly down.

Keep your shoulders relaxed and loose.

Keep your head straight and chin slightly down.

1

2

face with a slight smile. Keep your body weight distributed equally on both legs. Breathe naturally, but breathe in when your hands move up.

3 For Kicking With Feet (Right), bend both knees slowly until you have squatted about 20 degrees. Be sure to keep your knees over your feet, but not past your toes, as you bend them. Breathe out slowly while bending your knees. Move both arms down and bend your elbows at the same time until your upper arms are alongside your body and there is about a 110-degree angle between your forearms and upper arms. Keep your neck, head, and upper body straight; keep your shoulders relaxed and loose; and keep your body weight equally distributed between both legs. Shift your body weight gradually onto your left leg. Slightly turn your upper body to the right as you start a downward circular path to bring your arms to the front of your body. Move your head slightly down so as to be able to follow the movement of your right hand as it creates a circular path. Practice steps 2 and 3 together several times to give yourself a good sense of control over your balance at the beginning of this form.

4 Cross your hands parallel to the ground in front of you at your waist, with both palms turned toward your body and your left hand on top. Start shifting your body weight onto your left leg. Keep your neck, head, and upper body straight and your shoulders relaxed and loose. Keep your knees bent. Look straight ahead.

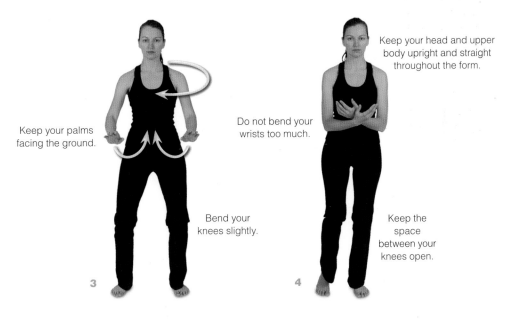

Keep your palms facing the ground.

Do not bend your wrists too much.

Bend your knees slightly.

Keep your head and upper body upright and straight throughout the form.

Keep the space between your knees open.

5 Shift your body weight entirely onto your left leg. Move your right foot slightly in toward your left leg and raise your right leg so that only your right toes touch the ground. Raise both hands in front of your chest at the same time as you move your right leg. Practice this movement several times to get a sense of security when your weight is entirely on one leg.

(continued)

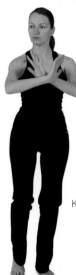

Keep your left knee bent.

Move slowly when
shifting weight.

5

6 **To kick right, keep
moving your hands and arms
up. Then separate them in
front of your face, with your
right hand moving forward,
palm facing out, and your left
hand moving to the left and
slightly back, palm facing
out. Move your left arm to
the back slightly to help you
remain balanced. Raise
your right knee straight up,
and at the same time kick
your right foot out slowly
while remaining in full
control of your balance.
The kicking and moving
the arms out happen
simultaneously. Have
the front leg in the same
direction of the kicking leg.**

Let your elbows
bend slightly.

At the apex of the kick, the
knee of the standing leg
and the knee of the kicking
leg are slightly bent.

Bend your ankle up to
strengthen the kick so
that it is a heel-first kick.

6

TIP Since one leg is moving while the other is slightly bent, static, and balancing all of your body weight, this movement can be challenging. You can
hold onto a chair on your left side and just practice the kicking movement
itself at first. When you feel that you can control the kicking movement, start
your kicking practice without the chair. You can begin kicking by only raising your leg slightly and kicking the lower part of the leg out a little, gradually increasing how high you raise your leg and how much you kick out.

7 To transition into Kicking With Feet (Left), bring your right leg down and place your right foot lightly on the ground, with your toes touching the ground first and then the rest of the foot. Shift your body weight gradually back onto your right leg until your body weight is equally distributed between both legs and move both hands down in front of your waist. Breathe naturally.

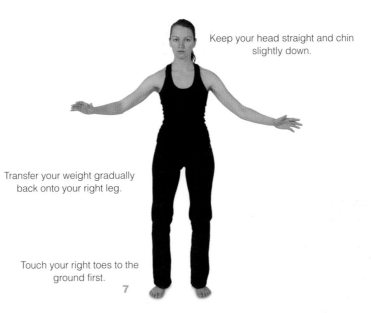

Keep your head straight and chin slightly down.

Transfer your weight gradually back onto your right leg.

Touch your right toes to the ground first.

7

8 For Kicking With Feet (Left), bend both knees slowly until you have squatted about 20 degrees. Be sure to keep your knees over your feet, but not past your toes, as you bend them. Breathe out slowly while bending your knees. Move both arms downward and bend your elbows at the same time until your upper arm is alongside your body and there is about a 110-degree angle between your forearms and upper arms. Keep your neck, head, and upper body straight; keep your shoulders relaxed and loose; and keep your body weight equally distributed between both legs. Shift your body weight gradually onto your right leg. Slightly turn your upper body to the left as you start a downward circular path to bring your arms to the front of your body. Move your head slightly down so as to be able to follow the movement of your left hand as it makes it circular path.

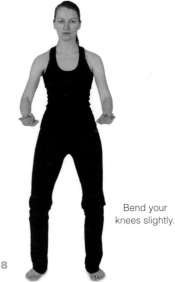

Bend your knees slightly.

8

(continued)

9 Cross your hands parallel to the ground at your waist, with both palms turned toward your body and your right hand on the top. Start shifting body weight onto your right leg. Keep your neck, head, and upper body straight and shoulders relaxed and loose. Keep your knees bent. Look straight ahead.

10 Gradually shift your body weight entirely onto your right leg. Move your left foot slightly in toward your right leg and raise your left leg so that only your left toes touch the ground. Raise both hands in front of your chest at the same time as you move your left leg. Practice this movement several times to get a sense of security when your weight is entirely on one leg.

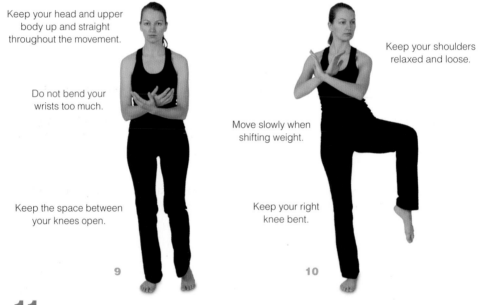

Keep your head and upper body up and straight throughout the movement.

Do not bend your wrists too much.

Keep the space between your knees open.

Keep your shoulders relaxed and loose.

Move slowly when shifting weight.

Keep your right knee bent.

9

10

11 To kick left, keep moving your hands and arms upward. Then separate them in front of your face, with your left hand moving forward, palm facing out, and your right hand moving to the right and slightly back, palm facing out. Move your right arm to the back slightly to help you remain balanced. Raise your left knee straight up, and at the same time kick your left foot out slowly while in full control of your balance. The kicking and moving the arms out happen simultaneously. Have the front leg facing the same direction as the kicking leg. When kicking, do not wholly straighten your kicking leg; your knee needs to be slightly bent even at the apex of the kick. Since one leg is moving while the other is bearing all your weight, this movement can be challenging. You can hold a chair on your right side and just practice the kicking movement itself at first. When you feel that you can control the movement, start your kicking practice without the chair. You can begin kicking by only raising your leg slightly and kicking the lower part of the leg out a little, gradually increasing how high you raise your leg and how much you kick out.

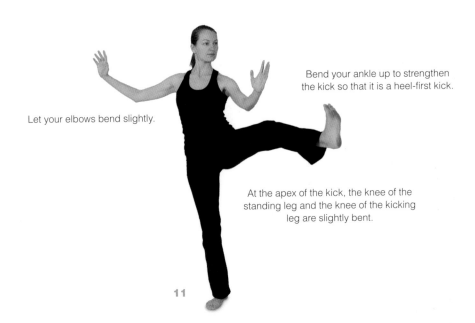

Let your elbows bend slightly.

Bend your ankle up to strengthen the kick so that it is a heel-first kick.

At the apex of the kick, the knee of the standing leg and the knee of the kicking leg are slightly bent.

11

12 To transition back to Kicking With Feet (Right), bring your left leg down and place your left foot lightly on the ground, touching the ground with the toes first and then the rest of the foot. Shift your body weight gradually back onto your left leg until your body weight is equally distributed between both legs, and move both hands down in front of your waist. Breathe naturally.

13 Repeat Kicking With Feet several times, alternating the kicking leg. Once you are ready to finish the movement, continue to step 14.

14 To close the form, shift your body weight back onto both legs equally. Move your arms up and out to shoulder level, with palms facing down and parallel to the ground (see figure *a*). Bring both arms down alongside your body and straighten your knees so that you are back in the starting position (see figure *b*). Breathe naturally and focus on your Dan Tian; breathe out when your hands move down.

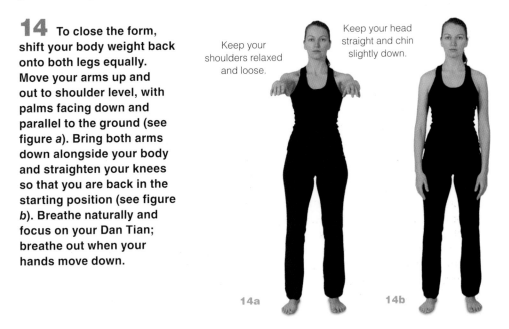

Keep your shoulders relaxed and loose.

Keep your head straight and chin slightly down.

14a

14b

Standing on One Leg (page 125)

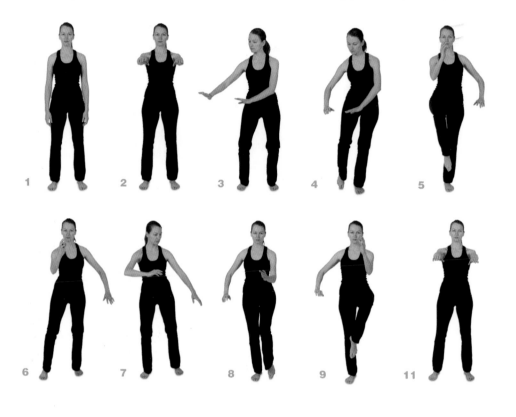

Kicking With Feet (page 130)

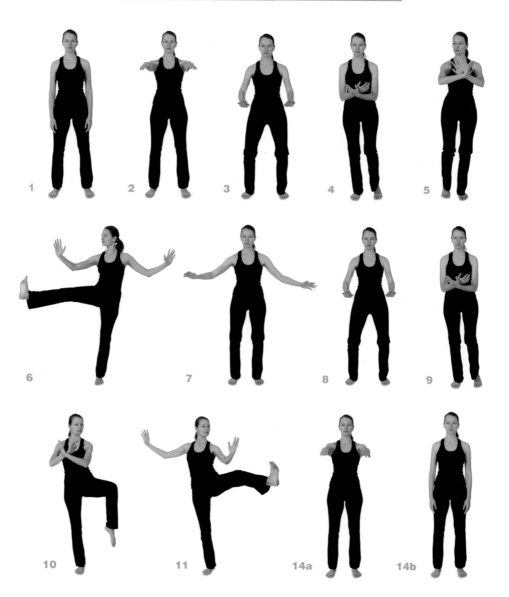

chapter 9

Forms for Coordination

Motor coordination ability, or simply coordination, is critical to daily life functions. Like other functions, coordination declines with age, and poor coordination can significantly affect quality of life. Fortunately, coordination can be improved through practice, and tai chi is an excellent exercise for improving coordination. This chapter introduces two tai chi forms that have been demonstrated to improve coordination. Improve your coordination, and improve the quality of your life!

Coordination, or to use a more scientific term, *neuromuscular coordination,* is the ability to organize and activate large and small muscles with the right amount of force in the most efficient sequence. In real life, coordination often refers to the ability to coordinate the eyes, hands, feet, and body so that a particular movement can accomplish a goal. Almost all daily life tasks, such as preparing food, writing, driving, and working in the yard, require some sort of coordination. When a physical task requires the integration of vision and hand movement, the coordination is sometimes called *eye–hand coordination.*

Similar to other aspects of the body, coordination is affected by aging. When we are young, few of us even notice the existence of coordination. However, as we get older and our coordination declines, we realize it is critical to our quality of life. As an example, many older adults have difficulty turning dials on appliances, using a paintbrush, or even performing simple cooking tasks. In the later years, many older adults even have difficulty making telephone calls, opening jars, and grasping, carrying, and placing objects around the house, which makes independent living almost impossible.

Fortunately, coordination can be improved with practice. A number of studies have shown that people can regain their coordination after systematic training. As an example, a 1984 study found that many excellent 60-year-old typists can type as fast as 20-year-old typists (Salthous, 1984). They do so by reading farther ahead in the text than younger typists so that they can anticipate the movements to be made. How can tai chi help improve coordination? Unlike the simple and straight movements in other physical activities, such as throwing and kicking, tai chi movements are acts of coordination—you must consistently move your body weight from one leg to another while your hands and other parts of the body coordinate simultaneously.

In this chapter, you will learn two tai chi forms designed specifically to improve coordination. The original movements of these forms require a rather large space. To help the beginner, the forms were modified so that you can practice in a space of 1 square yard or meter. Again, practice can be done anywhere, inside or outside. It is okay to practice while barefoot as long as the surface is safe for bare or stocking feet. You can start practicing the foot patterns, and after you feel comfortable with them, you can add the arm movements. Gradually, you will integrate all the movements and start to enjoy the smooth coordination of various parts of your body.

Practice tai chi and enjoy your new and improved coordination!

Level
▶ Beginner

Benefits
▶ Strengthens the legs.
▶ Strengthens the arms.
▶ Improves coordination.
▶ Improves body awareness.
▶ Improves shoulder, neck, and head health.
▶ Improves qi flow in hand meridians.

Contraindications
▶ Falling with loss of balance

Vega Working at Shuttles

Yu Nu Quan Suo

The name of this form derives from its movement pattern. A shuttle is a weaving tool designed to neatly hold the weft thread while weaving. The shuttle is passed back and forth between the warp threads as they raise and lower, making a tunnel of sorts that the shuttle passes through. The movements of this form, led by the arms, are similar to someone weaving with two shuttles, moving gently and constantly in a circle from left to right and then right to left. In addition, because of the martial arts origin of tai chi, the form is also an offensive move—while one arm blocks an opponent's arms or fists, the other arm strikes while moving your body forward.

TIP To perform Vega Working at Shuttles correctly, coordinate hand and leg movements with weight shifting, but do not shift body weight until complete balance is achieved. Also, keep some distance between the legs to maintain better balance.

1 For the starting position, stand naturally with your legs shoulder-width apart and your feet parallel to each other. Keep your upper body, head, and neck upright and straight. Hold your chin slightly down and relax your face with a slight smile. Hang your arms down along your sides with your hands resting naturally beside your thighs. Keep your body weight equally distributed onto both legs. Clear your mind and keep a peaceful mental state throughout the whole form.

2 Raise your arms slowly in front of your body until they are level with your shoulders; your arms will be parallel to each other, shoulder-width apart,

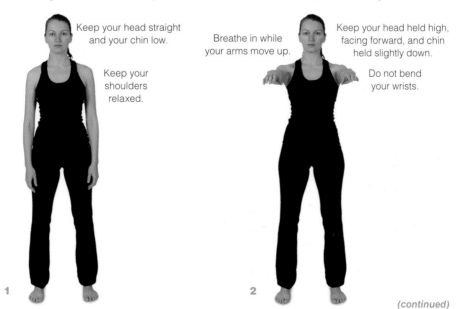

Keep your head straight and your chin low.

Keep your shoulders relaxed.

Breathe in while your arms move up.

Keep your head held high, facing forward, and chin held slightly down.

Do not bend your wrists.

1

2

(continued)

and your palms will be facing down. Keep your upper body, head, and neck straight. Hold your chin slightly down and relax your face with a slight smile. Keep your body weight distributed equally between both legs.

3 To shuttle left, shift the body weight to your right leg gradually, ending with your left toes touching the ground. Move your left hand down toward the front of your right side and turn your left palm up while you move your right arm slightly up to shoulder level. End the movement when you appear to be holding a large ball in front of your right side.

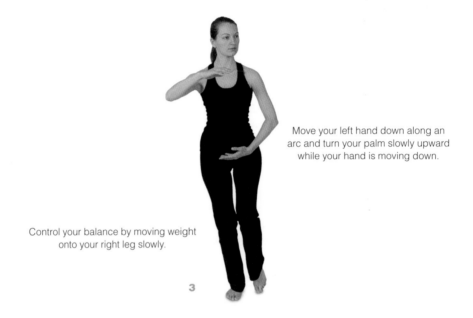

Move your left hand down along an arc and turn your palm slowly upward while your hand is moving down.

Control your balance by moving weight onto your right leg slowly.

3

4 To shuttle forward, move your left leg one step straight forward, with the heel touching the ground first and keeping most of your body weight on your right leg; move your left hand upward and right hand forward with palms facing out (see figure *a*); and start to shift your body weight onto your left leg, gradually ending with your entire left foot firmly on the ground. Meanwhile, keep moving your left hand up and right hand forward (see figure *b*). Finish shifting your body weight onto your left leg, ending in a left bow stance (your hands and the leg in bow stance should point in the same direction) with your left hand just above your left temple, palm turned obliquely up, and your right hand pushed forward in front of the midline of your body; keep looking forward to maintain your stability and balance; and make sure both heels are on parallel lines with about a foot (30 cm) between the lines (see figure *c*).

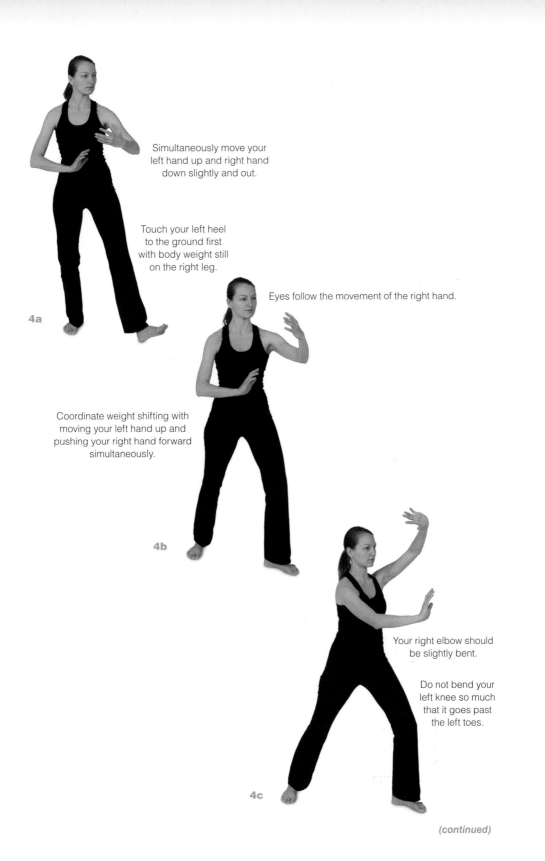

Simultaneously move your left hand up and right hand down slightly and out.

Touch your left heel to the ground first with body weight still on the right leg.

4a

Eyes follow the movement of the right hand.

Coordinate weight shifting with moving your left hand up and pushing your right hand forward simultaneously.

4b

Your right elbow should be slightly bent.

Do not bend your left knee so much that it goes past the left toes.

4c

(continued)

5 To transition from left to right, shift your body weight gradually back onto your right leg, raise your left toes with your left heel remaining on the ground, swivel your left foot to the right about 90 degrees, and slowly return your left toes to the ground. Meanwhile, move your left hand to the right with palm facing the ground while your right hand moves down with palm facing up (see figure *a*). End the transition by moving all of your body weight onto your left leg and raising your right heel so that only the right toes are on the ground. You should look like you are holding a ball in front of your left side (see figure *b*).

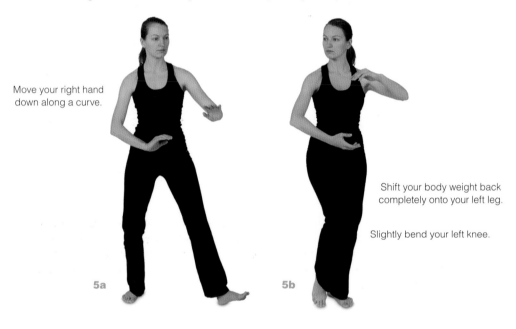

Move your right hand down along a curve.

5a

Shift your body weight back completely onto your left leg.

Slightly bend your left knee.

5b

6 To shuttle right, move your right leg one step straight forward with your heel touching the ground first, keeping most of your body weight on your left leg (see figure *a*); move your right hand upward and your left hand forward, palm facing out; and start to shift your body weight onto your right leg, gradually ending with your entire right foot firmly on the ground. Meanwhile, keep moving your right hand up and your left hand forward. Finish shifting your body weight onto your right leg, ending in a right bow stance (your hands and the leg in bow stance should point in the same direction) with your right hand just above your right temple, palm turned obliquely up, and left hand pushed forward in front of the midline of your body; keep looking forward to maintain your stability and balance; and make sure both heels are on parallel lines with about a foot (30 cm) between the lines (see figure *b*).

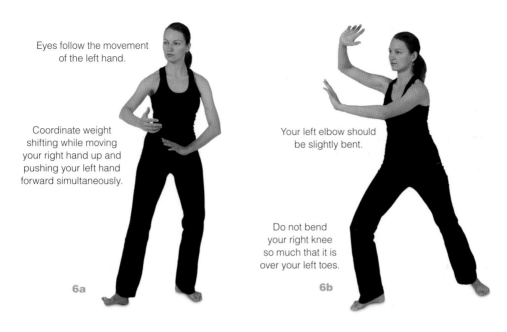

Eyes follow the movement
of the left hand.

Coordinate weight
shifting while moving
your right hand up and
pushing your left hand
forward simultaneously.

Your left elbow should
be slightly bent.

Do not bend
your right knee
so much that it is
over your left toes.

6a

6b

7 Repeat steps 3 through 6 several times. Once you are ready to finish the movement, continue to step 8.

8 To close the form, turn your body toward the front and shift your body weight equally onto both legs. Move your arms up and out to shoulder level, with your palms facing down and parallel to the ground. Bring both arms down alongside your body and straighten your knees as you lower your arms so that you are back in the starting position.

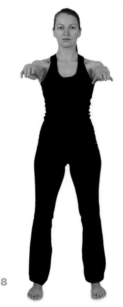

8

Cloud Hands

Yun Sou

The name of this form also derives from its movement pattern. During this form, your arms alternately rotate in front of your body, looking like clouds floating by. As a result, the movement is called *Waving Hands Like Cloud*, or more simply, Cloud Hands. The hand movement is the same as the movement you learned for Outside Vertical Circular Movement in Sequence in chapter 4, in which your hands also move along two circles in sequence in front of your body, with your right hand moving clockwise and your left hand moving counterclockwise. In the original martial arts context, the movement is used to block an opponent's continuous attack.

TIP Use your lumbar spine (low back) as the axis of your movement (i.e., your hand movement should follow your waist movement) and coordinate your weight shifting with your hands. Keep your hands within a comfortable distance from the body, neither too close nor too far; they should be at a distance where they can move comfortably along clockwise and counterclockwise circles. (Note that the hand movements are the same as Outside Vertical Circular Movement in Sequence on page 52 of chapter 4).

1 For the starting position, stand naturally with your legs shoulder-width apart and your feet parallel to each other. Keep your upper body, head, and neck upright and straight. Hold your chin slightly down and relax your face with a slight smile. Hang your arms down along your sides with your hands resting naturally beside your thighs. Keep your body weight equally distributed between both legs. Clear your mind and keep a peaceful mental state throughout the whole form.

2 Raise your arms slowly in front of your body until they are level with your shoulders; your arms will be parallel to each other, shoulder-width apart, and your palms will be facing down. Keep your upper body, head, and neck upright and straight. Hold your chin slightly down and relax your face with a slight smile. Keep your body weight distributed equally between both legs.

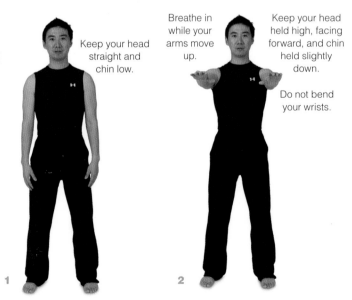

Keep your head straight and chin low.

Breathe in while your arms move up.

Keep your head held high, facing forward, and chin held slightly down.

Do not bend your wrists.

3 To shift weight to the right leg, turn your body slightly to the left, moving your right hand up and then down from right to left and then up along a clockwise circle (see figure *a*); face your palm toward yourself and follow your right hand with your eyes; shift your body weight onto your right leg in time with your right hand movement (see figure *b*); and move your left hand down along a counterclockwise circle (i.e., in an opposite direction) and follow the movement of your right hand in sequence (see figure *c*).

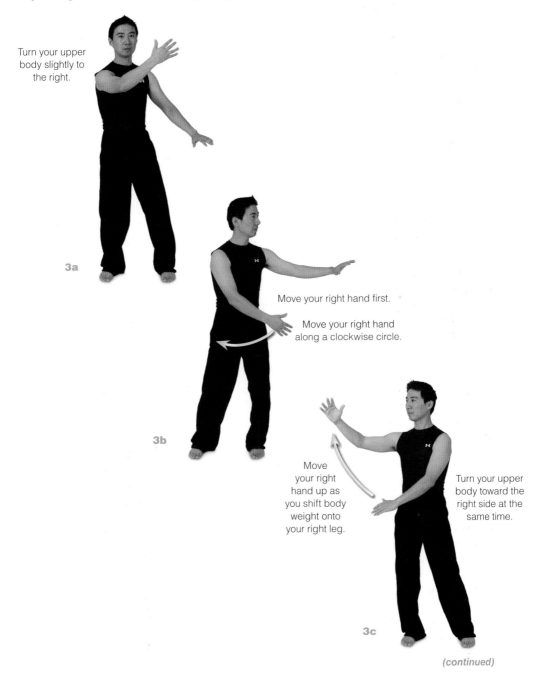

Turn your upper body slightly to the right.

3a

3b

Move your right hand first.

Move your right hand along a clockwise circle.

Move your right hand up as you shift body weight onto your right leg.

Turn your upper body toward the right side at the same time.

3c

(continued)

4 To shift your weight to the left leg, keep moving your right hand down along its clockwise circle; start to move your left hand up along a counterclockwise circle; slightly raise your left foot (see figure *a*); slide your left foot out a half step to the left side (see figure *b*); keep moving your left hand up along the circle and start to move your body weight onto your left leg; face your left palm toward yourself, following your left hand with your eyes (see figure *c*); shift your body weight completely onto your left leg as your left hand moves up; turn your upper body to the left; and move your right hand down along a clockwise circle, ready to move up for the next circle.

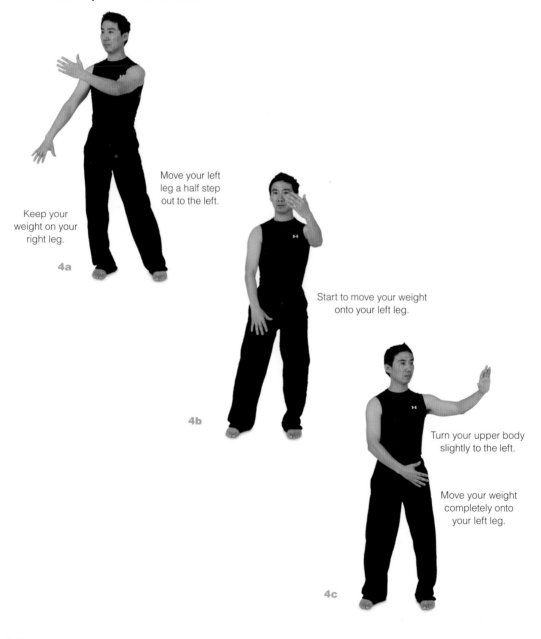

Move your left leg a half step out to the left.

Keep your weight on your right leg.

4a

Start to move your weight onto your left leg.

4b

Turn your upper body slightly to the left.

Move your weight completely onto your left leg.

4c

5 Repeat steps 3 and 4 several times. Once you are ready to finish the movement, continue to step 6.

6 To close the form, shift your body weight back onto both legs equally. Move your arms up and out to shoulder level with palms facing down and parallel to the ground (see figure *a*). Bring both arms down alongside your body and straighten your knees so that you are back in the starting position (see figure *b*).

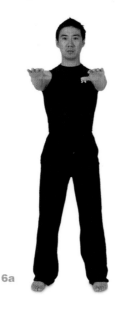
6a

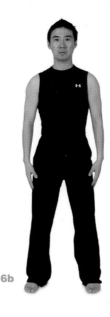
6b

Vega Working at Shuttles (page 141)

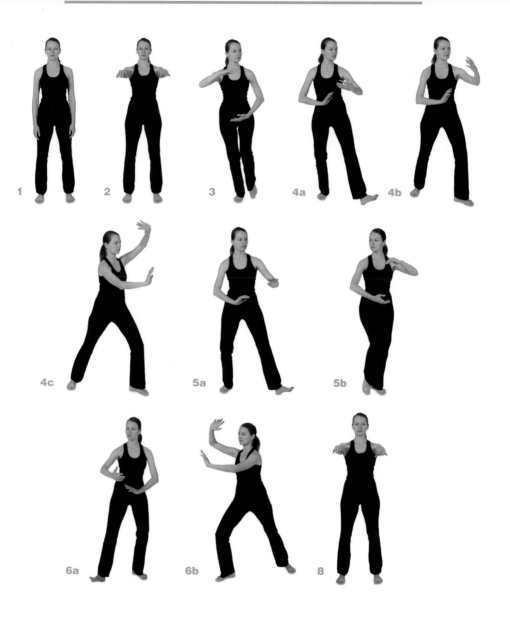

1

2

3

4a

4b

4c

5a

5b

6a

6b

8

Cloud Hands (page 146)

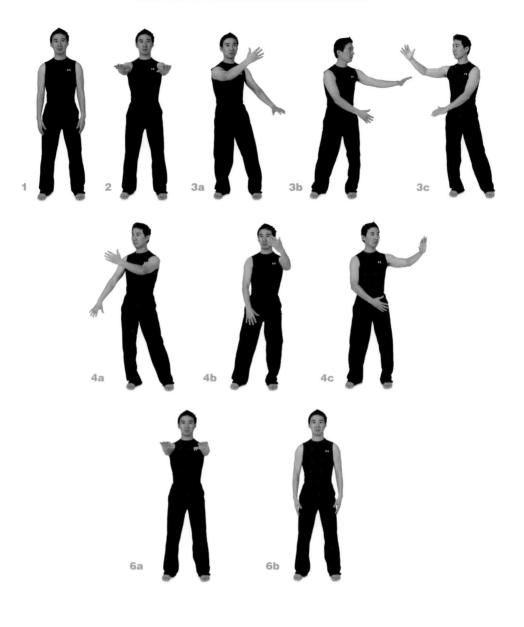

1

2

3a

3b

3c

4a

4b

4c

6a

6b

part III

Tai Chi Routines

Now that you have learned and practiced several tai chi forms, it is time for you to learn actual tai chi routines. A tai chi routine usually consists of a set of forms. A routine can contain as few as 6 forms (as in the routine you will learn in chapter 10) or as many as 108 forms. A tai chi routine is often developed by a specific tai chi school, which often has its own routines developed through many years of practice or by a panel of experts for public use. (The popular 24- and 48-form tai chi routines in China were developed by a panel specifically for public use.) Regardless of whether they are short or long, most tai chi routines include key movements and aspects of meditation. With a routine, teaching and learning tai chi become more fun and easier. In part III, three routines designed specifically for beginners are introduced in chapters 10 (a six-form routine), 11 (a twelve-form routine), and 12 (a push hands routine).

Practice and enjoy!

chapter 10

Six-Form Routine

In this chapter, you will learn an introductory six-form routine consisting of the following forms: Cloud Hands, Single Whipping, Playing Lute, Brush Knee and Twist Step, Parting Mustang's Mane, and Grasp Sparrow's Tail. You learned Cloud Hands in chapter 9, Brush Knee and Twist Step and Parting Mustang's Mane in chapter 6, and Grasp Sparrow's Tail in chapter 7. You will now learn two new forms, Single Whipping and Playing Lute, and integrate them with the other four forms into a set routine. Note that we purposely use the word *integrate* rather than *combine,* emphasizing that a routine is not simply a combination of individual tai chi forms. Rather, these forms integrate together to achieve a higher level of tai chi practice. Forms in this context are like individual pearls, which are beautiful alone, but when strung together as a necklace, they become greater—more beautiful, meaningful, and valuable.

Moving in a smooth, continuous manner at a consistent speed is the key to a good tai chi routine. Although forms are still done one by one in a routine, their individual existence should not stand out or be sensed by you. Rather, the forms integrate into a new, continuous, whole movement in which the end of one form is the beginning of the next. Smooth connections among forms, therefore, are critical when performing a routine. There are several ways to achieve smooth movement: Keep a constant, slow speed throughout, even during transitions from one form to another; make sure to finish each form completely (beginners often rush to start the next form instead of making a distinction between forms); and have a relaxed mind while at the same time paying attention to your performance of the routine.

Because a tai chi routine is designed to be practiced independently (e.g., the start of the routine acts as a warm-up and the closing as a cool-down), it can be practiced without combining it with other exercises, although some quick stretches and a few minutes of stance practice beforehand are helpful. A tai chi routine can also be practiced with other exercises (e.g., as part of cooling down after walking or other moderate- to high-intensity exercise).

Level
 ► Beginner

Benefits
 ► Strengthens the upper body.
 ► Strengthens the legs.
 ► Improves the cardiovascular system.
 ► Helps with stress management and low-back health.
 ► Improves coordination.
 ► Improves body awareness.
 ► Improves qi flow.

Contraindications
 ► Falling with loss of balance

1 Stand naturally with your legs together as you start this routine. Keep your upper body, head, and neck upright and straight (see figure *a*). Hold your chin slightly down and relax your face with a slight smile. Hang your arms down along your sides with your hands resting naturally beside your thighs. Take a small step outward with your left foot so that your feet are shoulder-width apart and your feet parallel to each other (see figure *b*). Keep your body weight equally distributed between both legs. Clear your mind and maintain a peaceful mental state throughout the whole form.

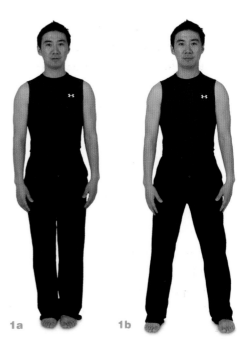

1a   1b

2 Maintain the starting position but raise your arms slowly in front of your body until they are at shoulder level. Your arms should be parallel, held shoulder-width apart, and palms should face down.

3 Slowly squat while simultaneously moving both arms down to the level of your waist. Keep your upper body upright while squatting slightly, with your knees going out toward your toes.

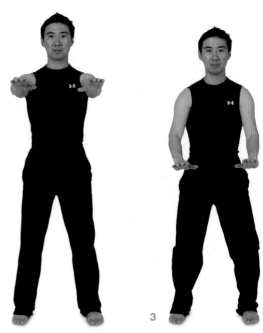

2   3

Cloud Hands

You learned the movement of Cloud Hands previously on page 146 of chapter 9. Make sure your foot movement follows a side-step pattern.

4 To shift your weight to your right leg, turn your body slightly to the left; move your right hand up and then down from right to left and then up along a clockwise circle; face your right palm toward yourself, following your right hand with your eyes; shift your body weight onto your right leg in time with your right hand movement; and move your left hand down along a counterclockwise circle (i.e., the opposite direction of your right hand's movement) and follow the movement of your right hand in sequence.

5 Keep moving your right hand down along its clockwise circle and start to move your left hand up along a counterclockwise circle. Slightly raise your left foot and slide your left foot out a half step to the left; most of your body weight should still be on your right leg.

6 To shift your weight onto your left leg, keep moving your left hand up along the counterclockwise circle and start to move your body weight onto your left leg, facing your left palm toward yourself and following your left hand with your eyes.

7 Shift your body weight completely onto your left leg as your left hand is moving up, turn your upper body toward your left side, move your right hand down along its clockwise circle, move your right leg a half step toward your left leg, and land your right foot lightly beside your left foot.

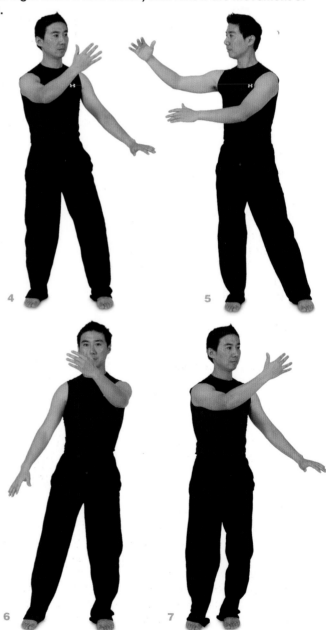

Single Whipping

The name of this form derives from its movement: One hand moves in an arc while the other is pushed forward in a movement similar to cracking a whip. The form harkens back to its original martial arts purpose as a defensive and offensive move. One hand pushes forward to block an opponent's attack and start forward momentum to fight back as the back hand makes an arc in order to fight or to be in a ready position for fighting.

8 Turn your body to the right; shift your body weight gradually back onto your right leg; keep moving your left hand up; extend your right hand up and move your right arm back into a slightly cocked position, turning your palm toward the ground; and watch your right hand with your eyes.

9 Move your body weight completely onto your right leg; raise your left heel and get ready to move your left leg; keep moving your left hand up as you form a hook (hand form learned in chapter 4) with your right hand by bringing all the fingers together, touching each other at a single point with an empty space inside your palm; bend your right wrist; and end with your right arm at shoulder level.

10 Start to turn your body to the left; take a half step to the left with your left foot, with your left heel touching the ground first; keep almost all of your weight on your right leg; and keep moving your left hand up as it starts to pass your face.

11 To complete the Single Whipping, shift your body weight onto your left leg while bending your left knee so as to be in a left bow stance (about 70 percent of your weight should be on your left leg and 30 percent on your right leg); meanwhile, rotate your left palm slowly from facing you to facing away and push it forward on your left side, ending with your fingertips at eye level.

(continued)

Shifting your body weight onto your left leg and pushing your left hand and arm forward should be coordinated with each other. At the end of the Single Whipping, keep your right upper arm slightly below shoulder level and have about a 15-degree bend at the elbow, with your forearm being the higher part of your arm at around shoulder level, and hold your left elbow directly above your left knee with your left arm slightly bent. Look forward over your left hand.

Playing Lute

The lute was a popular stringed musical instrument in ancient China. Since the movement of this form is similar to playing a lute, it was named accordingly.

12 Shift your body weight completely onto your left leg and start to move your right foot a half step forward toward your left heel; pull your left hand down and back slightly and move your right hand forward.

13 Land with your right foot behind your left heel, continuing to move your left hand up and your right hand down. When moving your left hand up, the movement should be leftward, upward, and forward following a circular path; when moving your right hand down, the movement should be coordinated with the body weight shifting back onto your right leg.

14 Shift body weight back onto your right leg, with your left toes lifting off the ground and your knee slightly bent to make a left empty step, and turn your left hand up while following a circular path at about nose level, with your left palm facing right and your left elbow slightly bent. Meanwhile, move your right hand to the inside of your left elbow with your palm facing left, and end the movement when you are in a posture that looks similar to playing a lute. Look forward with your eyes just over the top of your left fingertips.

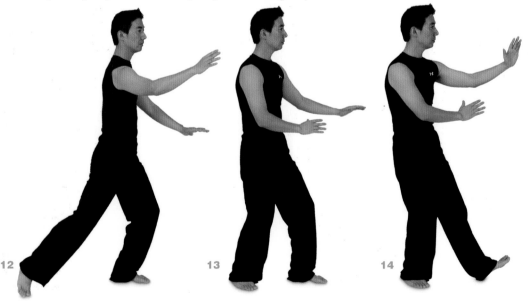

12   13   14

Brush Knee and Twist Step

You learned the movement of Brush Knee and Twist Step previously on page 89 of chapter 6.

15 Move your body weight onto your right leg; turn your upper body 90 degrees to the right; turn your right hand so that the palm is facing up and move your right arm up; turn your left hand so that the palm is facing down while you are turning your right hand so that the palm is facing up, and move your right arm down and then up; take a half step back with your left leg, ending with your left toes touching the ground; and watch your right hand with your eyes.

16 Take a full step to the left with your left leg, touching the ground with your left heel first (see figure *a*) and then placing the whole foot down (see figure *b*); turn your upper body to the left and push your right hand straight out at ear level; move your left hand over your left knee; and end the movement with your legs in a left bow step (make sure there are about 12 in. or 30 cm between the feet when in a bow step), with your right arm reaching straight out, palm facing out, and your left hand facing the ground at waist level on the left side of your knee (see figure *c*). While moving into the bow step, execute the left and right hand movements simultaneously and move your face, front foot, and pushed-out hand in the same direction.

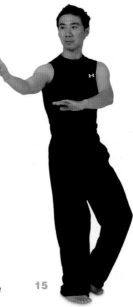

15

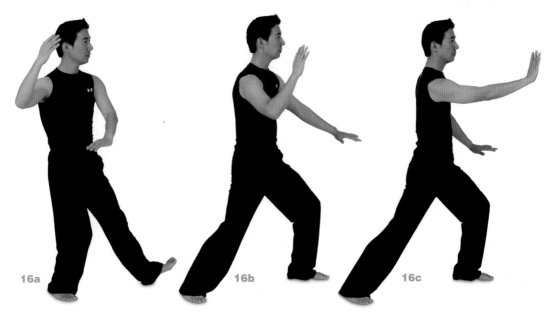

16a   16b   16c

Parting Mustang's Mane (Right)

You learned the movement of Parting Mustang's Mane (Right) previously on page 84 of chapter 6.

17 Move your body weight back onto your right leg; turn your left foot about 45 degrees to the left; turn your upper body to the right; move your right hand down along a circle while you move your left hand up (see figure *a*); shift your body weight gradually back onto your left leg; keep moving your right hand down along the circle; raise your right foot almost completely off the ground to be ready to move forward (see figure *b*); move your body weight completely onto your left leg, move your right foot a half step forward, and stop at the instep of your left foot with your right toes slightly touching the ground; and turn your left hand over so that your left palm is facing the ground while you simultaneously turn your right palm so that it is facing your left palm, as if you were holding a large ball on the left side of your body (see figure *c*).

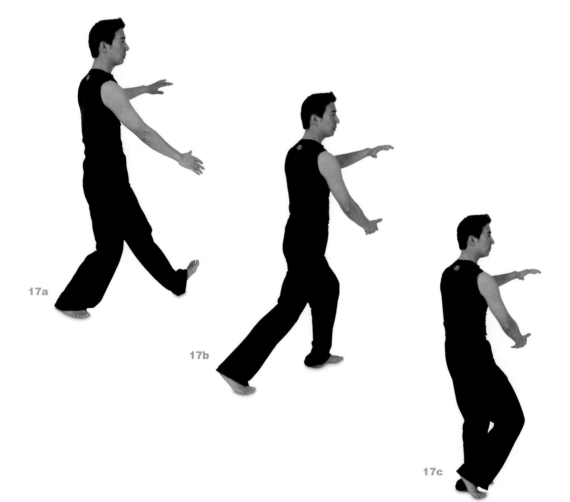

17a

17b

17c

18 To complete the form, take a full step with your right leg to the right, with your heel touching the ground first (see figure *a*); move your body weight gradually onto your right foot; move your right arm up and your left arm down; and end the movement with your right hand in front of your body, with your palm facing you, and your left hand alongside your left hip (see figure *b*).

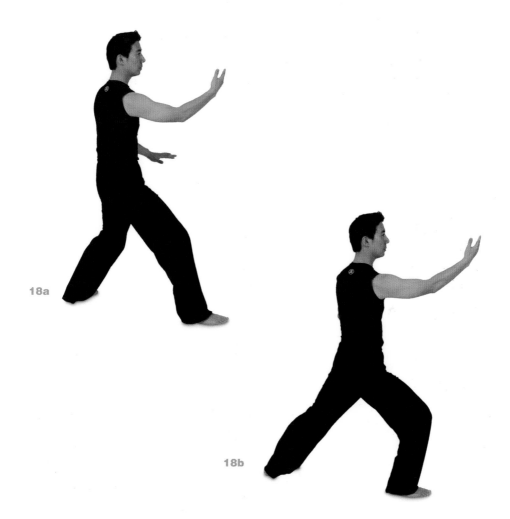

18a

18b

Grasp Sparrow's Tail

You learned the movement of Grasp Sparrow's Tail previously on page 109 of chapter 7.

19 Slightly move your body weight back onto your left leg; turn your right foot 45 degrees to the right while moving your right hand back and turning your palm 180 degrees to face the ground at the same time (see figure *a*); turn your left hand up simultaneously so it faces your right hand; shift your weight forward almost entirely onto your right leg while raising your left leg slightly with the knee bent (see figure *b*); and then transfer all your weight onto your right leg as you bring your left leg in close to your right leg, placing only your left toes on the ground. Meanwhile, move your left hand up and right hand down into the familiar holding-ball position in front of the right side of your body (see figure *c*).

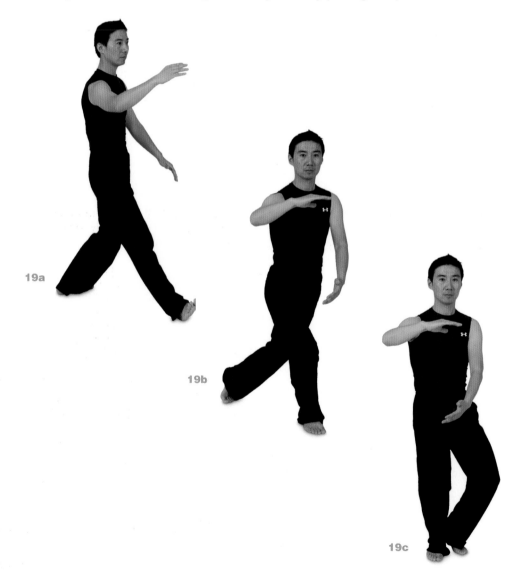

19a

19b

19c

20 With your left leg, take a full step to the left, with the heel touching the ground first (see figure *a*) and arms parallel to each other and the ground in front of your body, and shift your body weight gradually onto your left leg, ending in a left bow step. Meanwhile, push your left arm upward and forward along a curve and press your right hand down, ending at waist level with the palm facing the ground (see figure *b*).

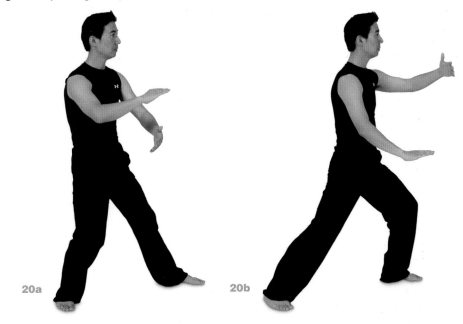

20a   20b

21 Turn both palms so that they are facing each other (see figure *a*), and pull both hands back and down together to your right front while shifting your body weight back onto your right leg (see figures *b* and *c*).

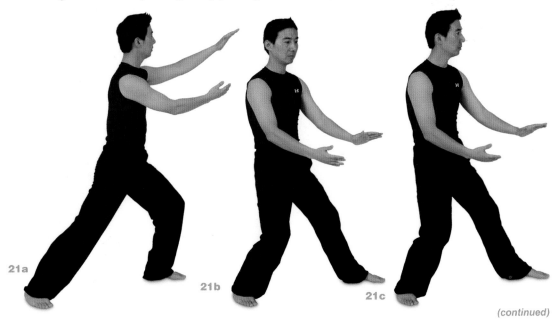

21a   21b   21c

(continued)

22 Turn your left palm toward yourself and your right palm away from you. With your palms touching, move your left hand forward by pushing it with your right hand (see figures *a* and *b*) while shifting your body weight onto your left leg, ending in a left bow step (see figure *c*).

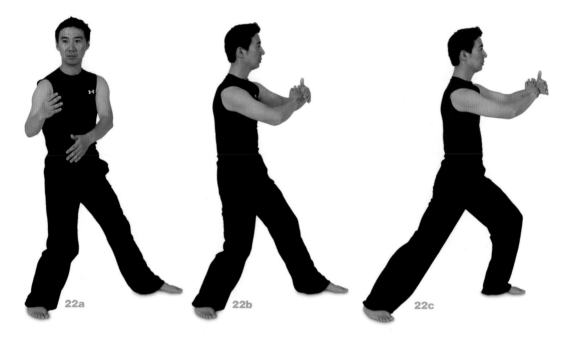

22a   22b   22c

23 Release both hands by pushing them forward, with palms facing the ground (see figure *a*). Shift your body weight back onto your right leg and raise your left toes so that only your left heel is on the ground while you pull both hands back into your body (see figure *b*).

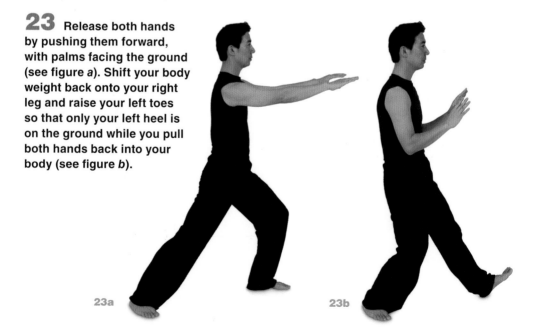

23a   23b

24 Push both hands down, shift your body weight forward onto your left leg (see figure *a*), and end in a left bow step with both hands out in front of you at just below shoulder level with palms pushing out (see figure *b*).

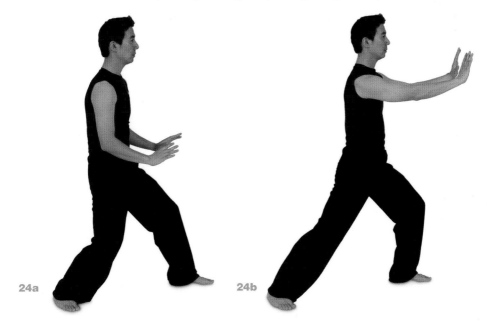

24a   24b

Closing With Cross Hands

This is a closing form in which you first separate your arms while turning your body back to the starting direction and then cross your hands in front of your chest, forming an *X*. The ending position gives it its name.

25 Turn your body to the right while moving your weight onto your right leg and pivot on your left heel so that your left toes move inward. Move your right hand in an even arc from your left side to your right side, passing in front of your face and away from your left hand.

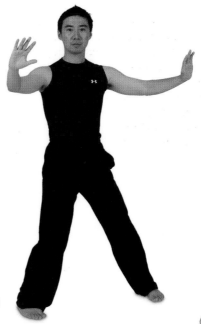

25

(continued)

26 Bend both knees while moving both hands down along an arc from outside to inside.

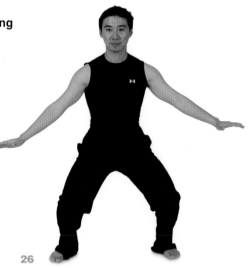

26

27 Cross both hands in front of your abdomen, with your right hand on the outside and both palms facing you (see figure *a*), and stand up gradually. Raise your crossed hands to chest level and take a half side step with your left leg toward your right leg (see figure *b*). Raising your body, taking a half side step, and crossing your hands should occur simultaneously.

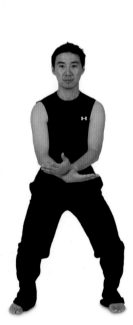

27a

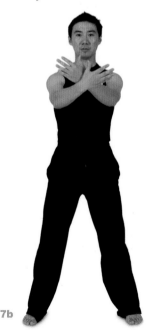

27b

28 Stand up straight with your body weight distributed evenly between both legs, and separate your hands in front of your chest, with both palms facing down (see figure *a*). Move your arms down (see figure *b*), move your left leg a half step toward your right leg so that both feet are together, and move your arms to the relaxed, natural, hanging starting position (see figure *c*).

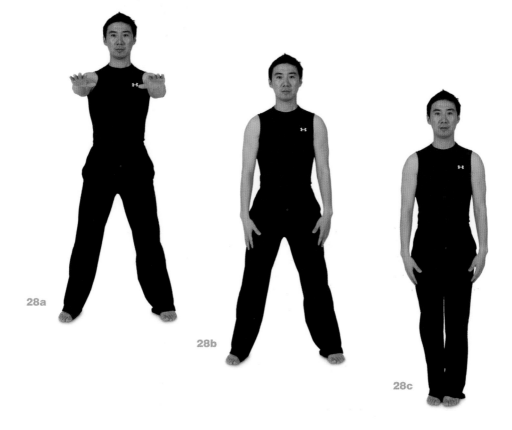

28a

28b

28c

According to the custom of Chinese martial arts, including tai chi, one should return to the starting position when finishing a routine. To do that for the Six-Form Routine you just finished, you can follow what is called the *duplication* or *complementary* form of the routine. This form is the same as the one you just learned, but it is executed in the opposite direction with the left and right sides switched (in other words, they are a mirror image). When you finish practicing these forms, you should be able to return to the starting position naturally. You can also simply repeat the Six-Form Routine several times to get similar health benefits.

Six-Form Routine

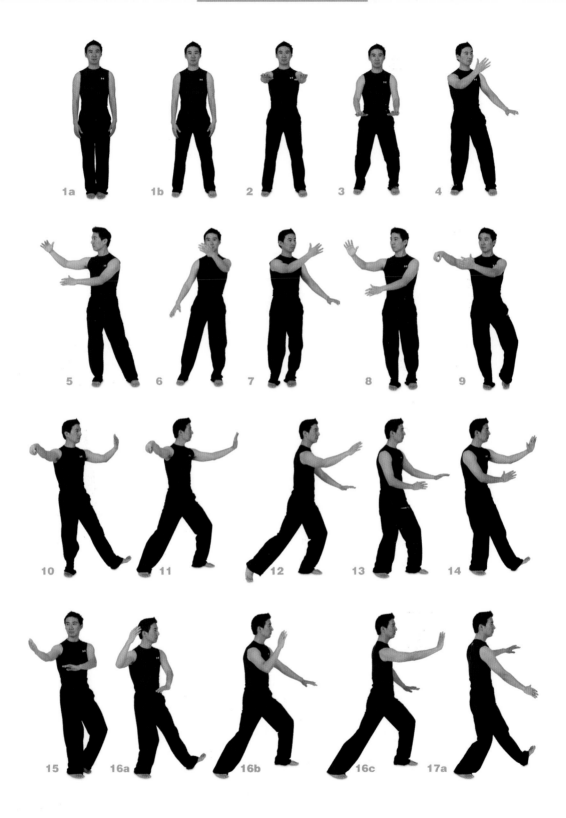

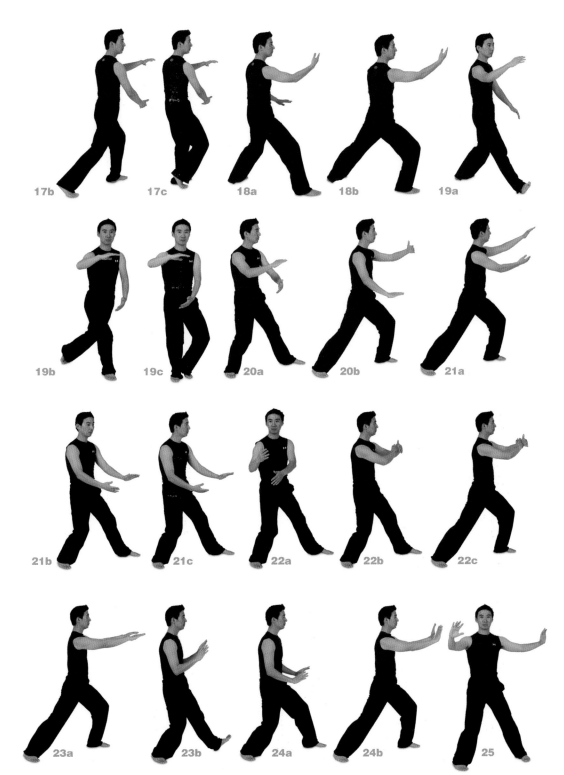

17b　　17c　　18a　　18b　　19a

19b　　19c　　20a　　20b　　21a

21b　　21c　　22a　　22b　　22c

23a　　23b　　24a　　24b　　25

(continued)

Six-Form Routine

(continued)

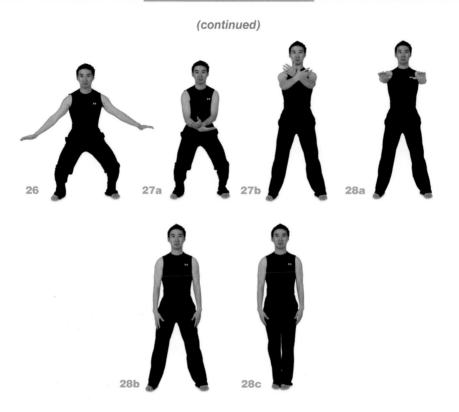

26 27a 27b 28a

28b 28c

chapter 11

Twelve-Form Routine

After learning the Six-Form Routine in chapter 10, you have a basic understanding of what a routine is and can start to enjoy the flow of tai chi. Expanding from the Six-Form Routine, you will now learn the Twelve-Form Routine in this chapter. The first part of the Twelve-Form Routine is the same as the Six-Form Routine, except that Closing With Cross Hands moves to the end of the entire routine. The rest of the forms in the second part of this routine are also forms you are familiar with because they are ones you learned in the previous chapters, and one of the forms is actually from the Six-Form Routine but is performed twice—Grasp Sparrow's Tail.

The 12 forms in this routine are as follows:

Cloud Hands	Deflect, Parry, and Punch (Right)
Single Whipping	Kicking With Feet (Left)
Playing Lute	Standing on One Leg
Brush Knee and Twist Step	Vega Working at Shuttles
Parting Mustang's Mane (Right)	Grasp Sparrow's Tail (Right)
Grasp Sparrow's Tail (Left)	Closing With Cross Hands

Pay attention to the transitions between forms and make sure one form flows smoothly into the next. The keys to helping the flow of the routine that were described in chapter 10 are also applicable here: Keep a constant, slow speed throughout the routine, even during transitions from one form to another; make sure to finish each form completely (beginners often rush, starting the next form instead of making a distinction between forms); and have a relaxed mind while at the same time paying attention to your performance of the routine. You should master the Six-Form Routine first, and then while learning the Twelve-Form Routine you can add new forms gradually so as not to feel overwhelmed.

The best way to learn a routine is to follow an instructor. For self-learning, it is perfectly all right to stop during the routine to check this book or the video clips prepared for the book. Practice with a partner (or partners) where you take turns reading the instructions aloud while doing the routine. Practice in front of a full-length mirror if available. Relax while doing the routine; feel and enjoy the flow that it generates. Practice every day if possible, or at least three times a week. Repeat the routine two to three times each time you practice. Since most of the important tai chi forms have been included, you can simply repeat the routine rather than doing the opposite-side directions, or mirroring the forms, as was recommended for the Six-Form Routine.

Level
▶ Beginner

Benefits
▶ Strengthens the upper body.
▶ Strengthens the legs.
▶ Improves the cardiovascular system.
▶ Helps with stress management.
▶ Helps maintain low-back health.
▶ Improves coordination.
▶ Improves body awareness.
▶ Improves qi flow.

Contraindications
▶ Falling with loss of balance

1 Stand naturally with your legs together as you start this routine. Keep your upper body, head, and neck upright and straight. Hold your chin slightly down and relax your face with a slight smile. Hang your arms down along your sides with your hands resting naturally beside your thighs (see figure *a*). Take a small step outward with your left foot so that your feet are shoulder-width apart and your feet parallel to each other (see figure *b*). Keep your body weight equally distributed between both legs. Clear your mind and maintain a peaceful mental state throughout the whole form.

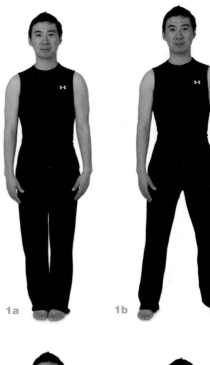

1a   1b

2 Maintain the starting position but raise your arms slowly in front of your body until they are level with your shoulders; your arms will be parallel, held shoulder-width apart, and palms will be facing down.

3 Slowly squat while moving both arms down simultaneously to waist level. Keep your upper body upright while squatting slightly, with your knees bending in the direction of your toes.

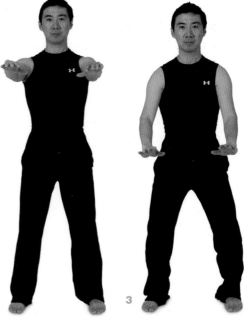

2   3

Cloud Hands

You learned the Cloud Hands form on page 146 of chapter 9. Make sure your foot movement follows a side-step pattern.

4 To shift your weight onto your right leg, turn your body slightly to the left; move your right hand up and then down from right to left, then up along a clockwise circle, with your right palm facing yourself and your eyes following your right hand; shift your body weight onto your right leg in time with your right hand movement; and move your left hand down along a counterclockwise circle (i.e., the opposite direction of your right hand movement) and follow the movement of the right hand in sequence.

5 Keep moving your right hand down along its clockwise circle and start to move your left hand up along a counterclockwise circle, and slightly raise your left foot and slide it out a half step to the left. Most of your body weight should still be on your right leg after you complete the left half side step.

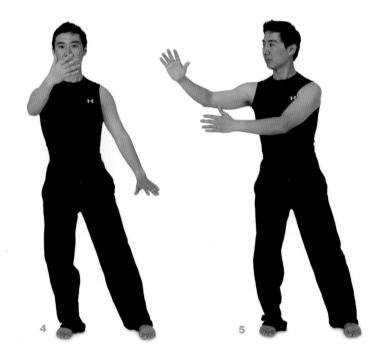

6 To shift your weight onto your left leg, keep moving your left hand up along the counterclockwise circle and start to move your body weight onto your left leg, with your left palm facing yourself and your eyes now following your left hand.

7 Shift your body weight completely onto your left leg as your left hand moves up, turn your upper body to the left, move your right hand down along its clockwise circle, move your right leg a half step toward your left leg, and land your right foot lightly alongside your left foot.

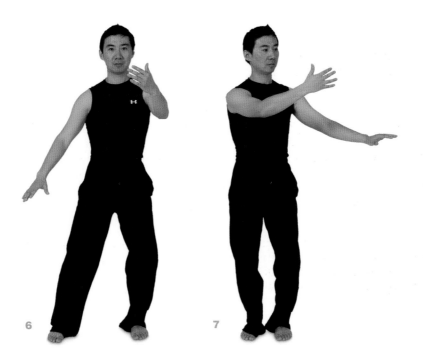

Single Whipping

You learned the Single Whipping form previously on page 159 of chapter 10.

8 Turn your body to the right; shift your body weight gradually back onto your right leg; keep moving your left hand up; extend your right hand up and move your arm back into a slightly cocked position, turning your right palm toward the ground; and watch your right hand with your eyes.

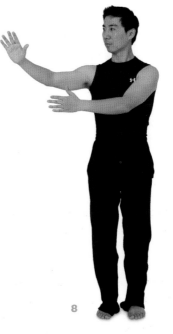

(continued)

Single Whipping *(continued)*

9 Move your body weight completely onto your right leg; raise your left heel and get ready to move your left leg; and keep moving your left hand up as your right arm moves out. All fingers of the right hand come together and touch each other at a single point, with an empty space inside your palm; bend your right wrist so that your right hand looks like a hook; and stop extending your right arm at shoulder level.

10 Start to turn your body to the left; take a half step using your left foot, with your left heel touching the ground first; keep almost all of your weight on your right leg; and keep moving your left hand up as it starts to pass your face.

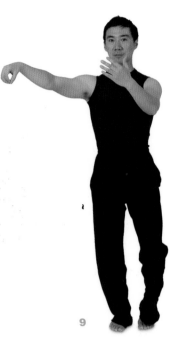

9

11 To complete the Single Whipping, shift your body weight onto your left leg while bending your left knee so that you are in a left bow stance (you should have about 70 percent of your weight on your left leg and 30 percent on your right leg). Meanwhile, rotate your left palm slowly from facing you to facing away and push it forward on your left side, ending with your fingertips at eye level. Look straight ahead past your left hand.

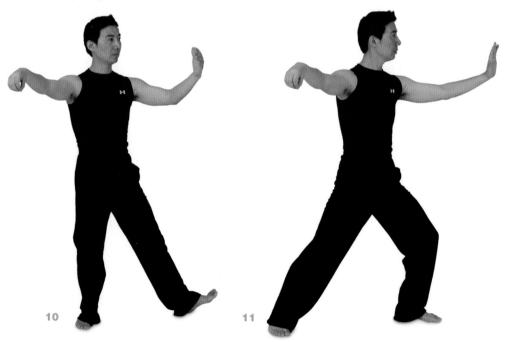

10

11

Playing Lute

You learned the Playing Lute form previously on page 160 of chapter 10.

12 Shift your body weight completely onto your left leg and start to move your right foot a half step forward toward your left heel; pull your left hand down and back slightly and move your right hand forward.

13 Land your right foot behind your left heel, and keep moving your left hand up and right hand down.

14 Shift your body weight back onto your right leg, with your left toes lifting up so that your left heel is still on the ground and your left knee slightly bent to make an empty step; turn your left hand up following a circular path at about nose level, with your left palm facing right and your left elbow slightly bent; meanwhile, move your right hand to the inside of your left elbow, with the palm facing left, and end the movement when you are in a posture that looks similar to playing a lute.

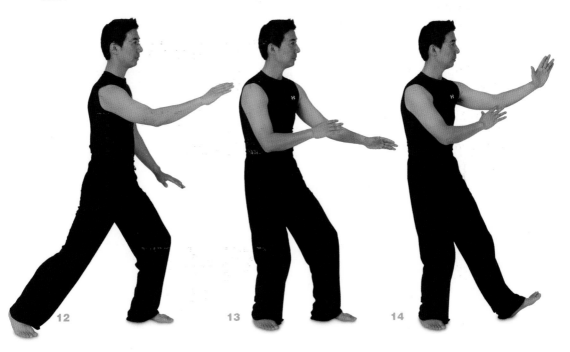

Brush Knee and Twist Step

You learned the Brush Knee and Twist Step form previously on page 89 of chapter 6.

15 Move your body weight onto your right leg; turn your upper body 90 degrees to the right; turn your right hand so that your palm is facing up and move your right arm up; turn your left hand so that your palm is facing down while you are turning your right hand so that the palm is facing up, and move your right arm down and then up; take your left leg slightly back, ending with your left toes touching the ground; and watch your right hand with your eyes.

16 Take a full step to the left with your left leg, touching the ground first with your left heel (see figure *a*) and then placing your whole foot down (see figure *b*); turn your upper body to the left and push your right hand straight out at ear level; move your left hand over your left knee; and end the movement with your legs in a left bow step, with your right arm reaching straight out, palm facing out, and your left hand facing the ground at waist level on your left side (see figure *c*).

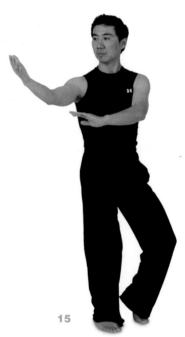

15

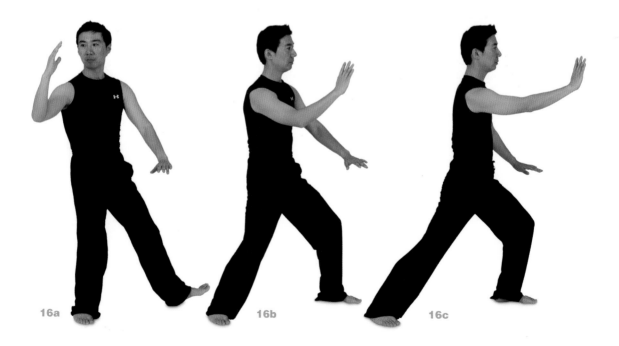

16a   16b   16c

Parting Mustang's Mane (Right)

You learned the Parting Mustang's Mane (Right) form previously on page 84 of chapter 6.

17 Move your body weight back onto your right leg; turn your left foot about 45 degrees to the left; turn your upper body to the right; move your right hand down along a circle while you move your left hand up (see figure *a*); shift your body weight gradually back onto your left leg; keep moving your right hand down along the circle; and raise your right foot almost completely off the ground to be ready to move forward (see figure *b*). Move your body weight completely onto your left leg and move your right foot a half step forward, stopping at the instep of your left foot with your right toes slightly touching the ground; and turn your left hand over so that your left palm is facing the ground while you simultaneously turn your right palm so that it is facing your left palm, as if you were holding a large ball on the left side of your body (see figure *c*).

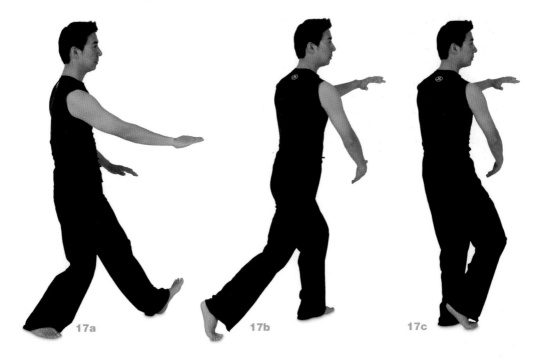

17a   17b   17c

(continued)

18 To complete the form, take a full step with your right leg to the right, with your heel touching the ground first; move your body weight gradually onto your right leg; move your right arm up and your left arm down (see figure *a*); and end the movement with your right hand in front of your body, palm facing you, and your left hand alongside your left hip (see figure *b*).

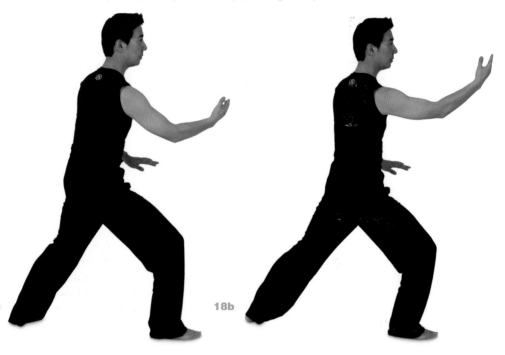

18a   18b

Grasp Sparrow's Tail (Left)

You learned Grasp Sparrow's Tail previously on page 109 of chapter 7.

19 Slightly move your body weight back onto your left leg; turn your right foot out 45 degrees to the right while moving your right hand back and turning your palm 180 degrees to face the ground at the same time; turn your left hand up simultaneously so that your left palm is facing your right palm (see figure *a*); shift your weight forward almost entirely onto your right leg while starting to raise your left leg slightly with the knee bent; and then transfer all your weight onto your right leg as you bring your left leg in close to your right leg and place only your left toes on the ground. Keep both knees bent, but body weight remains on your right leg only. Meanwhile, face your left hand up and right hand down into the familiar ball-holding position in front of the right side of your body (see figures *b* and *c*).

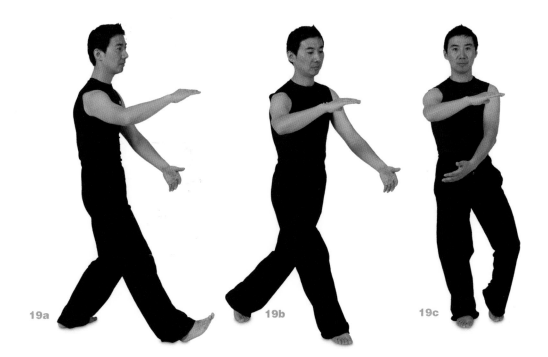

19a 19b 19c

20 With your left leg, take a full step to the left, with the heel touching the ground first and arms parallel to each other and the ground in front of your body (see figure *a*), and shift your body weight gradually onto your left leg, ending in a left bow step. Meanwhile, push your left arm upward and forward along a curve and press your right hand down, ending at waist level with the palm facing the ground (see figure *b*).

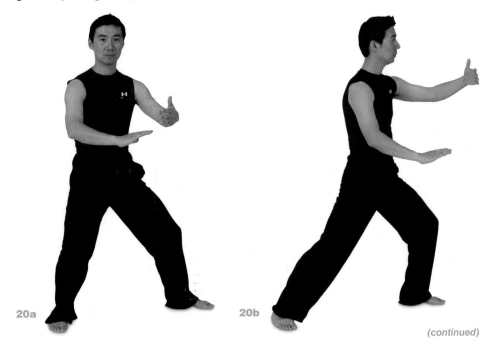

20a 20b

(continued)

21 Turn both palms so that they are facing each other (see figure *a*), and pull both hands back and down together to your right front while shifting your body weight back onto your right leg (see figures *b* and *c*).

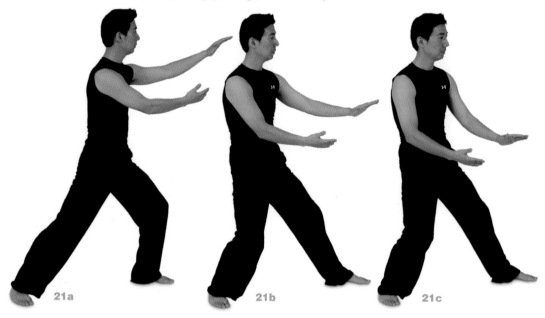

21a   21b   21c

22 Turn your left palm toward yourself and your right palm away from you. With your palms touching, move your left hand forward by pushing it with your right hand (see figures *a* and *b*) while shifting your body weight onto your left leg, ending in a left bow step (see figure *c*).

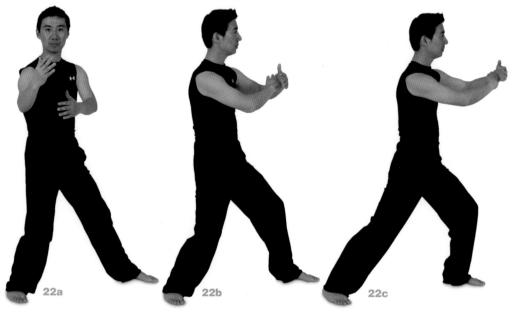

22a   22b   22c

23 Release both hands by pushing them forward, with palms facing the ground (see figure *a*). Shift your body weight back onto your right leg and raise your left toes so that only your left heel is on the ground while you pull both hands back into your body (see figure *b*).

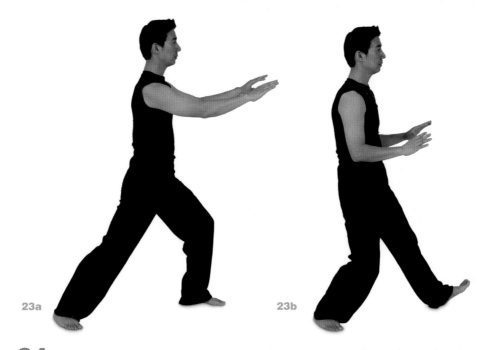

23a   23b

24 Push both hands down, shift your body weight forward onto your left leg (see figure *a*), and end in a left bow step with both hands out in front of you at just below shoulder level with palms pushing out (see figure *b*).

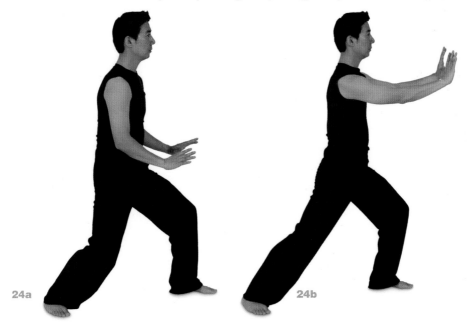

24a   24b

Deflect, Parry, and Punch (Right)

You learned the Deflect, Parry, and Punch form on page 115 of chapter 7.

25 Shift your body weight onto your right leg, turn your left foot about 45 degrees to the right, and turn your body and arms to the right at the same time.

26 Move your body weight back onto your left leg so that now your right leg has only the right toes touching the ground. Meanwhile, make a fist with your right hand and move it down along a vertical circle in front of body from right to left (clockwise), and move your left hand slightly up, from left to right, to the front of your chest.

27 Move your arms arcing out and forward while taking a full step forward with your right leg, with the right heel touching the ground first; gradually move your body weight onto your right leg and end in a right bow step; both hands follow the weight shift, ending with your right fist up and out and your left hand close to your right elbow; and your eyes watch your right fist throughout the movement.

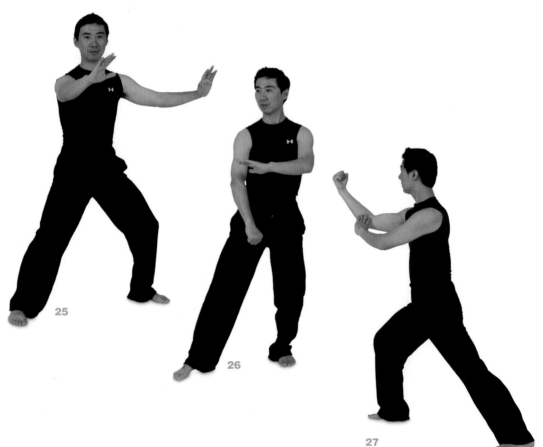

Kicking With Feet (Left)

You learned the Kicking With Feet form on page 130 of chapter 8.

28 Open your right fist while your left hand makes a counterclockwise horizontal ellipse that moves across the top of your right arm. An ellipse, as mentioned in chapter 8, is an unequal circle with one dimension longer than the other.

29 Open both hands in front of your chest by moving your left hand to the left and your right hand to the right; shift your body weight onto right leg at the same time.

30 Move your body weight completely onto your right leg and take a half step forward with your left foot, landing lightly by the instep of your right foot, with your left toes touching the ground. Bend your right knee slowly until it is bent about 20 degrees. Be sure to keep your knee over your foot, but not past your toes, as you bend it. Cross your hands parallel to the ground in front of your waist with both palms turned toward your body, your right hand on the top and closest to you. Keep your neck, head, and upper body straight and your shoulders relaxed and loose. Keep your knees bent. Look straight ahead.

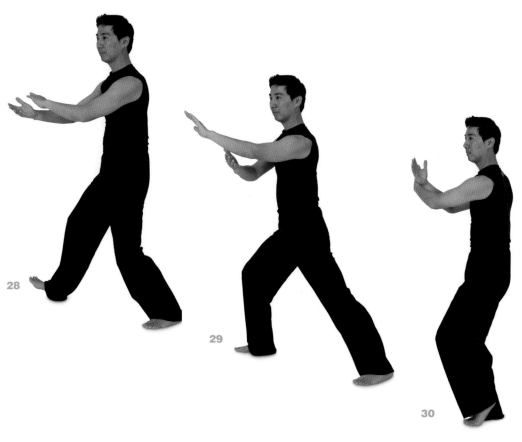

28

29

30

(continued)

31 Keep moving your hands and arms upward, separating them in front of your face with your left hand moving forward, palm facing out, and your right hand moving to the right and slightly back, palm facing out (your right arm moves to the back slightly to help you keep your balance). To kick left, raise your left knee straight up (see figure *a*) and at the same time kick your left foot out slowly while maintaining your balance (see figure *b*). When kicking, do not fully straighten your kicking leg; your knee needs to be slightly bent even at the apex of your kick. Because one leg is moving while the other is bearing all your weight, this movement can prove to be a challenge. You can reduce the difficulty by lowering your kicking leg and make sure you are in control of your balance before kicking.

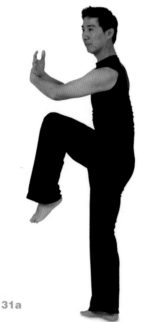

31a

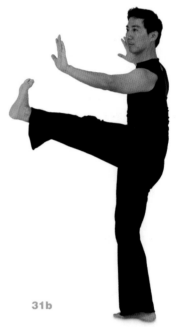

31b

Standing on One Leg

You learned the Standing on One Leg form on page 125 of chapter 8.

32 Return your left foot by bending your left knee (see figure *a*) and lightly landing your left foot parallel to your right foot (see figure *b*). At the same time, push your left hand down following a clockwise curve and move your right hand down slightly on the right side of your body.

33 Shift your body weight gradually onto your left leg and foot. Slightly turn your upper body to the right, lowering your arms and hands to waist level and keeping your palms parallel to the ground. Your right hand should be slightly in front of and above your right hip. Move your right hand, palm still facing the ground, in a slow clockwise circle. Tilt your head slightly downward so you can watch the path your hand is making.

34 Move all of your body weight onto your left leg. Raise your right leg slowly with your knee relaxed and bent. Raise your right hand at the same time at a slightly quicker speed than you are raising your right leg. Keep your left shoulder relaxed and slowly lower your left arm slightly. Use your left arm and hand to help you keep your balance. Keeping your left leg slightly bent also helps you keep your balance. Practice this part with great caution since it is easy to lose your balance when standing on only one leg.

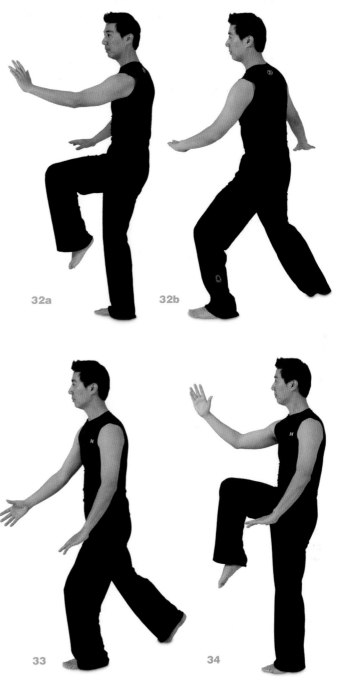

32a 32b

33 34

Vega Working at Shuttles

You learned the Vega Working at Shuttles form on page 141 of chapter 9.

35 Land your right foot naturally a half step in front of your body, and turn your body slightly to the right.

36 Shift your body weight onto your right leg, gradually ending with the toes of the left foot touching the ground. Move your left hand down toward the front of your right side, and turn your left palm up while you move your right arm slightly up to shoulder level. End in a holding-ball position in front of your right side.

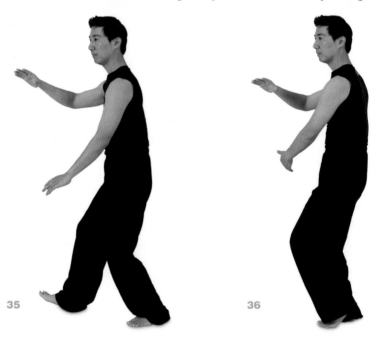

37 Move your left leg one step forward, touching the ground with your heel first and keeping most of your body weight on your right leg; move your left hand upward and your right hand forward with the palm facing out (see figure *a*); and start to shift your body weight onto your left leg, gradually ending with your entire left foot firmly on the ground. Meanwhile, keep moving your left hand up and your right hand forward (see figure *b*). Finish shifting your body weight onto your left leg, ending in a left bow stance with your left hand just above your left temple, palm turned obliquely upward, and your right hand pushed forward in the front of your midbody. Keep looking forward to maintain your stability and balance, and make sure both heels are on parallel lines with about 12 inches (30 cm) between the lines (see figure *c*).

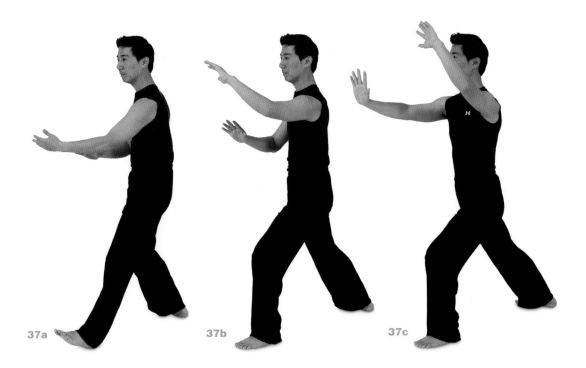

37a 37b 37c

Grasp Sparrow's Tail (Right)

You learned the movement of Grasp Sparrow's Tail on page 182 earlier in this chapter and also on page 109 of chapter 7.

38 Move your body weight back onto your right leg and turn your left foot slightly out to the left. Meanwhile, start to move your right hand down toward the front of your body and move your left hand down on the left side.

39 Shift your body weight almost entirely onto your left leg while raising your right leg slightly with the knee bent, bring your right leg in close to your left leg, and put only your right toes on the ground. Meanwhile, keep moving your left hand down toward the front of your body and turn your left palm down while you move your right arm down to shoulder level. End in the holding-ball position in front of your left side.

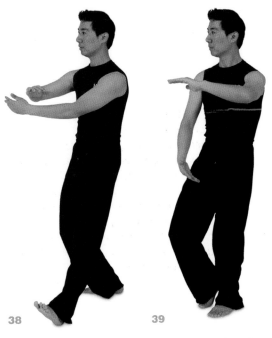

38 39

(continued)

Grasp Sparrow's Tail (Right) *(continued)*

40 Take a full step to the right with the right leg, touch your heel to the ground first while your arms are crossed in front of your body, and shift your body weight gradually onto your right leg, ending in a bow step. Meanwhile, push your right arm upward and forward along a curve and press your left hand down.

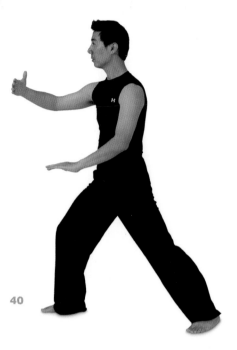

40

41 Turn both palms so that they are facing each other (see figure *a*) and pull both hands back and down together to your left front while shifting your body weight back onto your left leg (see figure *b*).

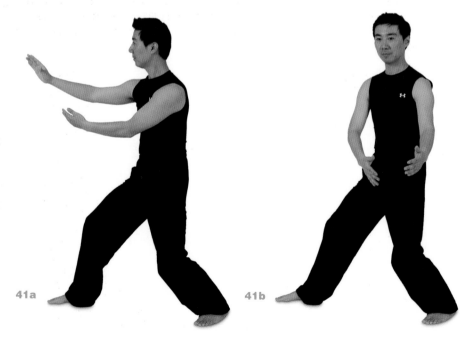

41a   41b

42 Turn your right palm toward yourself and your left palm away. With your palms touching, push your right hand forward using your left hand (see figure *a*) while shifting your body weight onto your right leg, ending in a right bow step (see figure *b*).

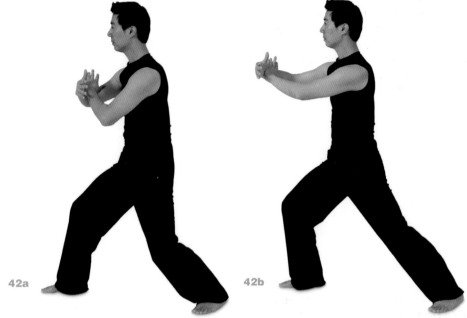

42a

42b

43 Release both hands by pushing them forward with your palms facing the ground (see figure *a*). Shift your body weight back onto your left leg and raise your right toes, with only your right heel touching the ground, while you pull both hands back into your body (see figure *b*).

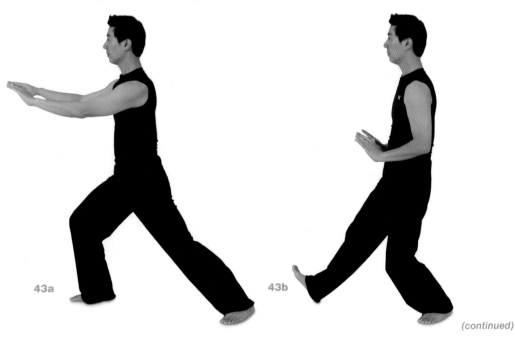

43a

43b

(continued)

44 Push both hands down, shift your body weight onto your right leg (see figure *a*), and end in a right bow step with both hands out, palms pushing outward (see figure *b*).

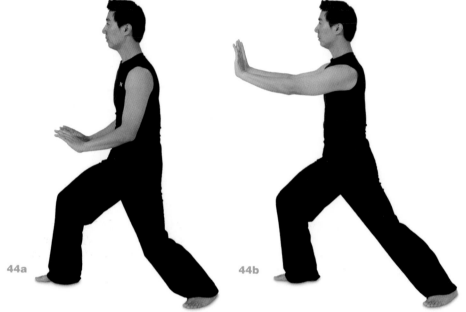

44a

44b

Closing With Cross Hands

The ending position of this movement gives it its name. You learned Closing With Cross Hands on page 167 of chapter 10 for the Six-Form Routine.

45 Turn your body to the left while moving your weight onto your left leg and pivoting your right toes inward. Move your left hand in an even arc from your right side to your left side, passing in front of your face and away from your right hand.

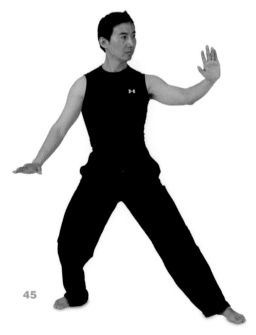

45

46 Bend both knees while moving both hands along an arc down from outside to inside.

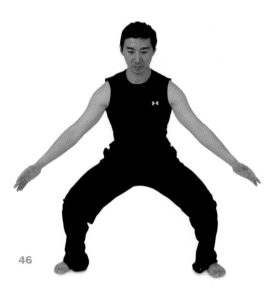

46

47 Cross both hands in front of your abdomen, with your right hand on the outside (see figure *a*) and both palms facing you. Stand up gradually, raising your crossed hands to chest level and taking a half side step with your left leg toward your right leg at the same time (see figure *b*).

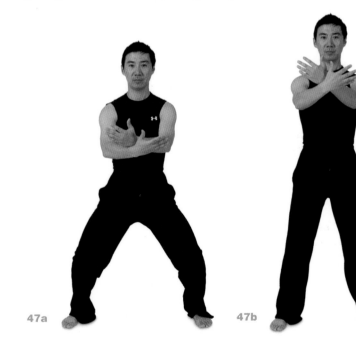

47a   47b

(continued)

48 Stand up straight with your body weight distributed evenly between both legs, and separate your hands in front of your chest, with both palms facing down (see figure *a*). Move your arms down (see figure *b*), move the left leg a half step toward your right leg so that both feet are together, and move your arms to the relaxed, natural starting position (see figure *c*).

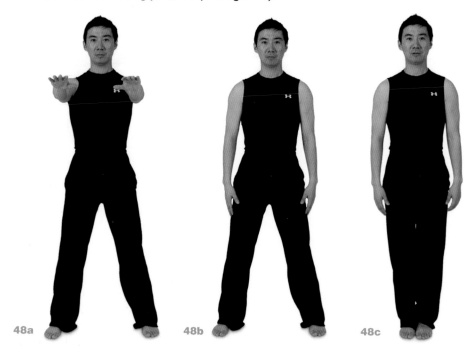

48a   48b   48c

Twelve-Form Routine

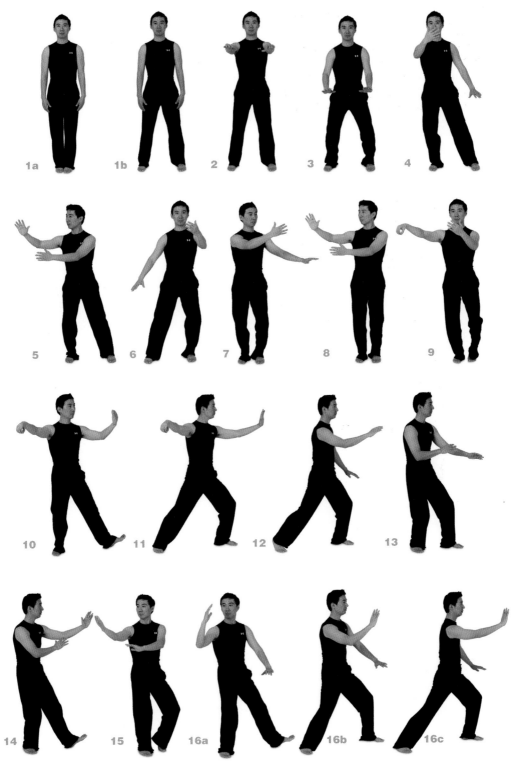

1a   1b   2   3   4

5   6   7   8   9

10   11   12   13

14   15   16a   16b   16c

(continued)

Twelve-Form Routine

(continued)

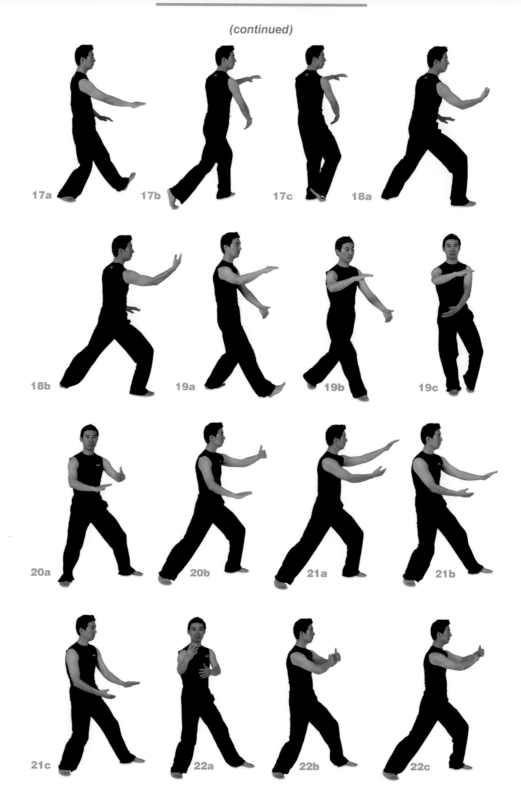

17a   17b   17c   18a

18b   19a   19b   19c

20a   20b   21a   21b

21c   22a   22b   22c

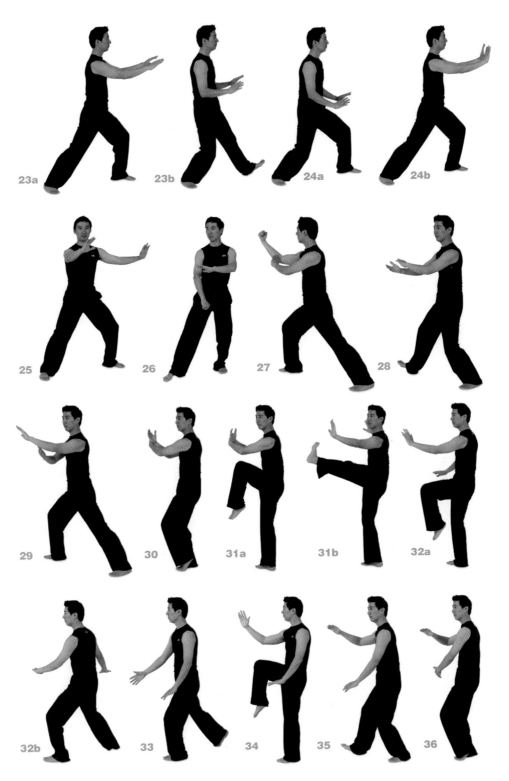

23a   23b   24a   24b

25   26   27   28

29   30   31a   31b   32a

32b   33   34   35   36

(continued)

(continued)

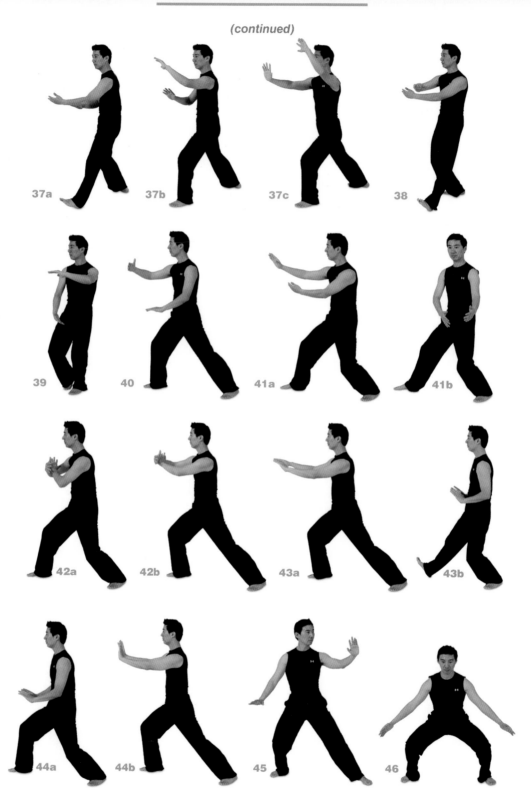

37a   37b   37c   38

39   40   41a   41b

42a   42b   43a   43b

44a   44b   45   46

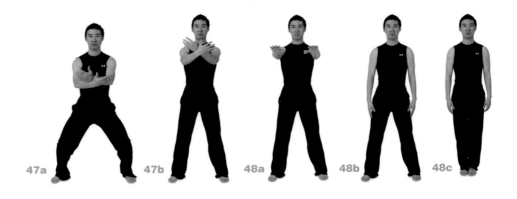

47a   47b   48a   48b   48c

chapter 12

Basic Push Hands Routine

Push hands is an advanced way to practice tai chi. Rather than practicing tai chi alone, as you did when learning the individual forms and routines in the earlier chapters, you must practice push hands with a partner. Remember that tai chi is rooted in martial arts, and push hands was originally required in order to learn how to apply tai chi in combat situations. As with tai chi forms and routines, most people learn and practice push hands for health and fitness purposes. Through push hands practice, you will be better able to understand the structure of tai chi movement techniques. More important, push hands practice will help you feel and experience the characteristics of tai chi strength: soft yet firm, an iron fist in a velvet glove. Finally, practicing push hands is the only way to experience the constant yin–yang changes generated in tai chi practice.

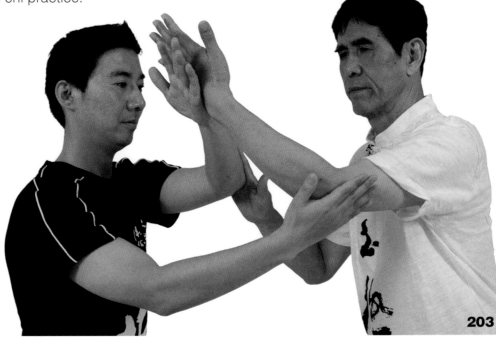

A major requirement for push hands practice is that both partners stand stable as they cross and touch each other's forearms. During practice, partners' arms remain in contact while moving without losing contact or hitting each other. Meanwhile, both partners constantly try to feel or locate each other's center of gravity so as to be able to move in a manner that could cause the other to lose his balance. In this way, you can gain control or win by using a small amount of strength and using your opponent's own strength against her or getting her to lose her balance. To counter this tactic, you can bend your knees more as you become stronger so that you have a more stable base, which will make it harder for your opponent to move you around.

Integrate push hands practice with the forms and routines learned in earlier chapters so that you gain a better understanding of the connections among them. The shifting of weight you learned in forms and routines, for example, is an important part of movement during push hands. Start with a partner at a similar skill level. You may feel helpless if you start your push hands practice with a partner who is more skilled than you; therefore, it is more fun to learn with a person at a similar level. Take your time to learn and enjoy tai chi. To understand the principle and beauty of push hands, you should practice each form step by step and learn to feel the strength of your partner.

In this chapter, you will learn and practice six basic push hands forms. Start by learning each form individually. After becoming familiar with them, you can start to integrate them into a practice. Specifically, you can do the appropriate form based on your opponent's move. To make the descriptions of movement easier to follow, we'll call the partners in the photos by the color they are wearing.

1 The partners (or opponents) stand facing each other about 4 to 5 feet (122-152 cm) apart.

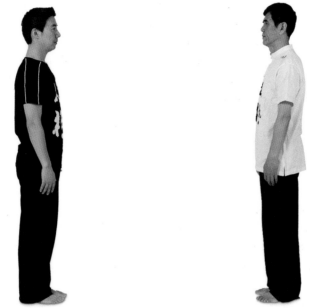

1

2 The partners start by separating their legs. The white partner moves his right leg and the black partner moves his left leg so that their legs are about shoulder-width apart.

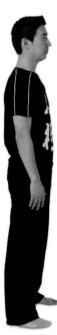

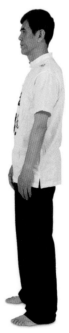

2

(continued)

(continued)

3 Both partners do the basic tai chi starting position and movement, raising the arms first (see figure *a*) and then lowering them (see figure *b*).

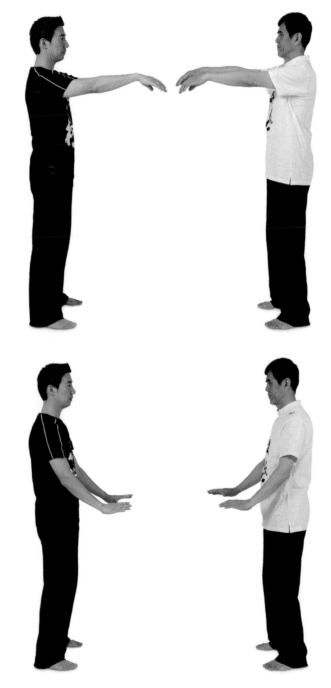

3a

3b

4 Both partners take one step forward with their right legs, raising and extending their right arms so that the backs of their right wrists touch each other.

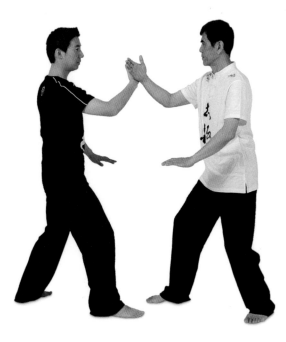

4

Horizontal Circle Pushing

The name of this form derives from its movement pattern, in which the movement of both partners' hands forms a horizontal circle.

1 The white partner starts to push forward using his right hand (see figure *a*) and shifts his body weight onto his front (right) leg at the same time (see figure *b*). The white partner needs to think of the black partner as a ball that must be hit in the center in order to deliver a hit that has full strength. Rather than pushing the white partner back directly, which violates the yin–yang (black partner–white partner) balance principle in tai chi, the black partner tries to guide the white partner to the right or left side. Maintaining the idea that the black partner is a ball, the black partner is trying to reduce the strength of the hit by having it hit off-center so as to roll off the ball (i.e., using his body, the black partner guides the white partner by feeling the direction of the white partner's pushing and moving his weight onto his back leg).

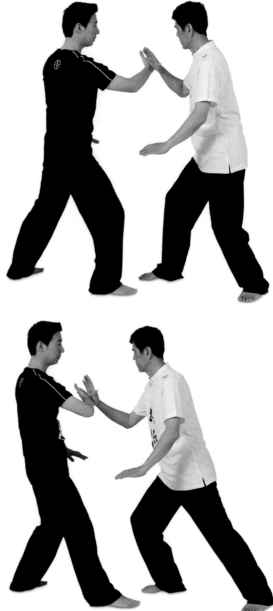

1a

1b

2 The black partner continues moving his weight back onto his back (left) leg and turns his body slightly to the right. At the same time, the black partner grasps the right elbow of the white partner with his left hand. There are two reasons for this: to prevent the white partner from using his elbow to hit the black partner's head and to help pull over the white partner using his own strength. The latter is one of the principles and beauties of tai chi in combat: Always use an opponent's strength against him.

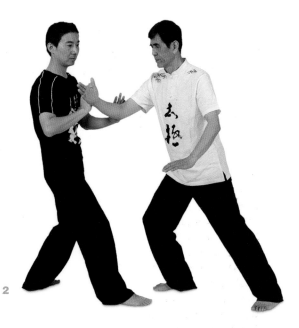

2

3 When the white partner feels that he will not hit the middle of the ball, so to speak, and there is a risk of losing his balance in continuing a forward movement, he pulls back his right arm and starts to move his weight onto the back (left) leg. The black partner, feeling the white partner pulling back, then starts to push forward so that he can take full advantage of the white partner's strength.

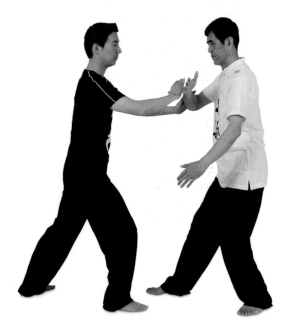

3

(continued)

4 As the white partner did in step 1, the black partner starts to simultaneously push forward and move his weight onto his front (right) leg (see figure *a*); meanwhile, the white partner tries to guide the black partner's hit to the right side of the ball (see figure *b*). The white partner now becomes a ball by moving his weight onto his back (left) leg and grasping the black partner's right elbow with his left hand to avoid being elbowed in the head.

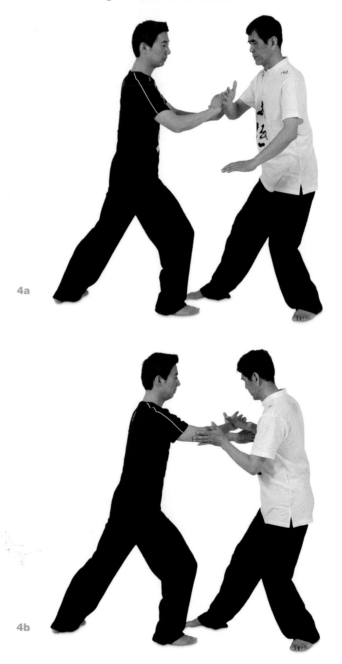

4a

4b

5 As in step 3, the black partner feels that he will not hit the middle of the ball and there is a risk of losing his balance, so he starts to pull back by moving his body weight onto his back (left) leg (see figures *a* and *b*). The white partner feels the black partner pulling back and starts to move forward, as in step 3.

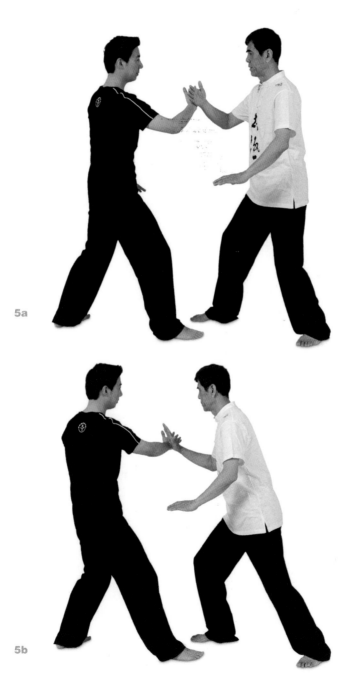

5a

5b

(continued)

6 Steps 1 through 5 can be repeated for the whole practice, or another form of push hands can be added to the practice. When a person hits (offense), he will try to hit the opponent's middle, and when he defends, he will try to lead the coming force to the side. When he finishes a hit and starts to pull back, his opponent starts to deliver his hit. Thus, during this push hands form the offense (yang) and defense (yin) continually repeat and continually switch which person is yang and which person is yin. The movement of both persons' hands forms a horizontal circle during this practice (see figures *a-f*).

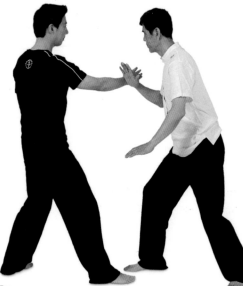

6a

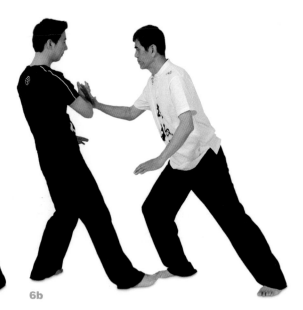

6b

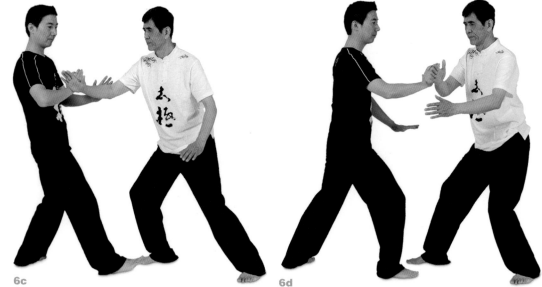

6c

6d

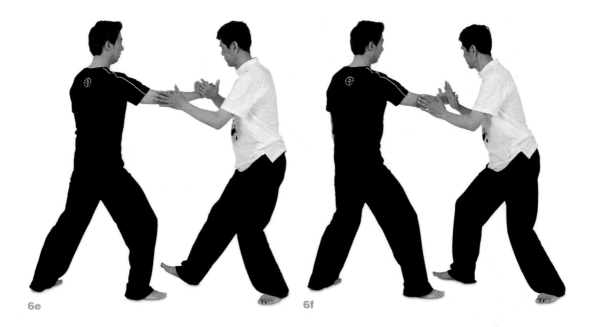

6e   6f

7 When finished, both partners move their right legs back to the front. Both reach out their arms and then lower them in a relaxed manner to the starting position.

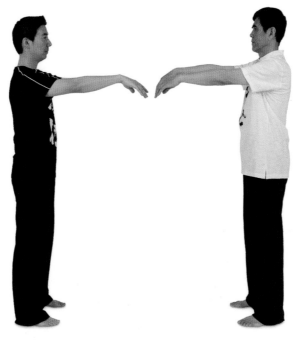

7

Horizontal Circle Bing Push Hands

You learned the *bing* movement on page 111 of chapter 7. Pushing an arm forward with the forearm in the front is called a *bing* in tai chi. In Horizontal Circle Bing Push Hands, therefore, you push back and forth with your forearms. Specifically, you form a circle using your arms in your front of your body, with your palms facing yourself without turning your wrists.

1 **The white and black partners stand facing each other 4 to 5 feet (122-152 cm) apart (see figure *a*). They start by separating their legs, the white partner moving his right leg and the black partner moving his left leg. Both take one step forward with their right legs, extending and crossing their right forearms so that the backs of their wrists touch (see figure *b*).**

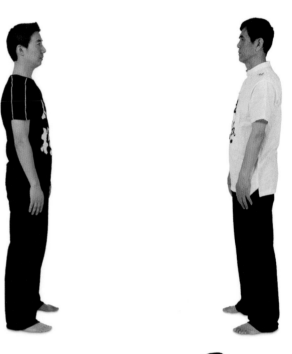

1a

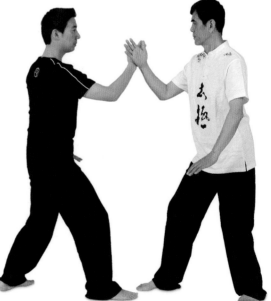

1b

2 Imagining the white partner as a ball, the black partner starts to push his right arm forward at the center of the white partner with a *bing* form as the black partner shifts his body weight onto the front (right) leg. The white partner tries to avoid the hit by guiding the black partner's move by bending his front arm back while moving his weight onto his back (left) leg (see figure *a*) and grasping the black partner's elbow with his left hand (see figure *b*).

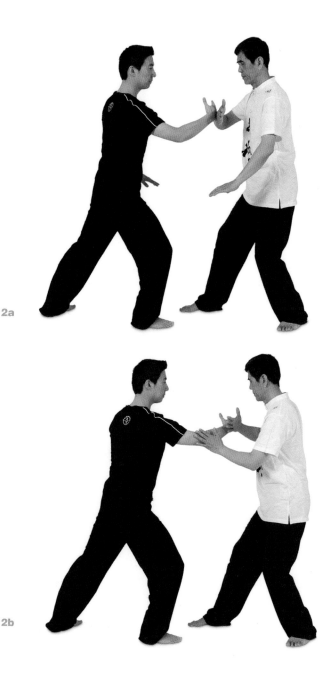

2a

2b

(continued)

3 When the black partner feels that he will not hit the center of the ball and there is a risk of losing balance in continuing forward movement, he pulls back his right arm as he starts to move his weight onto his back (left) leg. Feeling the black partner pulling back, the white partner starts to push forward to take advantage of the black partner's movement back.

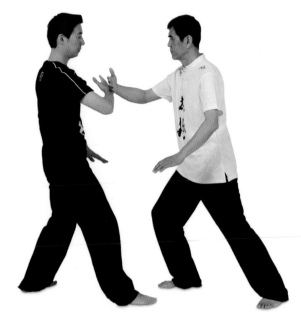

3

4 Similar to steps 2 and 3, the black partner avoids the white partner's hit by bending his arm, shifting his weight onto his back (left) leg, and grasping the white partner's right elbow using his left hand (see figure *a*). When he feels that he will not hit the white partner's center, the white partner pulls back, and at that moment, the black partner fights back by pushing forward.

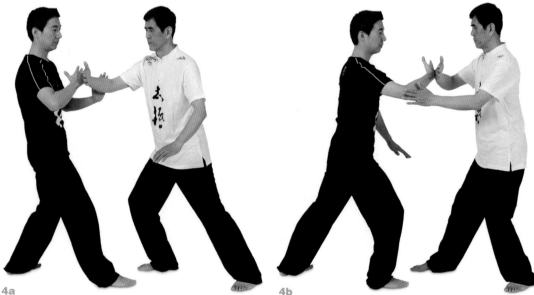

4a   4b

5 Steps 2 to 4 can be repeated for the entire practice.

6 When finished, both partners move their right legs back to the starting position. Both reach out their arms (see figure *a*) and then lower them in a relaxed manner to the starting position (see figure *b*).

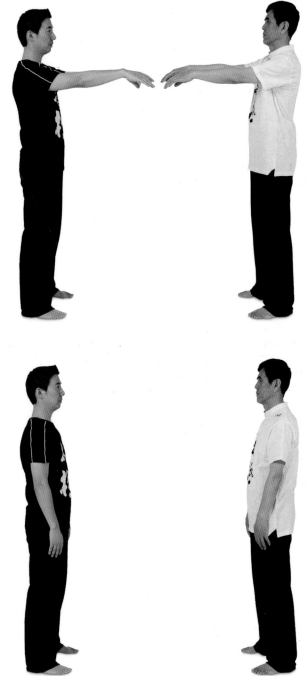

6a

6b

Vertical Circle Push Hands With Grasping

The name of this form reflects the key features of this push hands. *Vertical Circle* means the hands move in an up-and-down circle during the practice, while *Grasping* means that the partners grasp each other's hand and elbow during the practice to pull opponent toward one side and to avoid being elbowed.

1 The white and black partners stand facing each other about 4 to 5 feet (122-152 cm) apart. They start by separating their legs, the white partner moving his right leg and the black partner moving his left leg. Both take one step forward with the right leg, extending and crossing their right forearms so that the backs of their forearms touch.

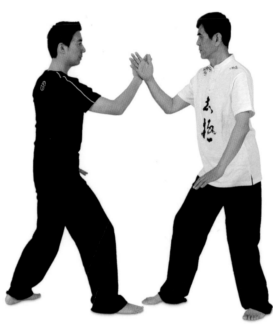

2 The black partner starts to push his right hand forward toward the white partner as he shifts his body weight onto his front (right) leg (see figure *a*). To deflect the hit by the black partner, the white partner guides the black partner's striking movement to the right and up by turning his body to the right, shifting his weight onto his back (left) leg and grasping the black partner's elbow with his left hand (see figure *b*).

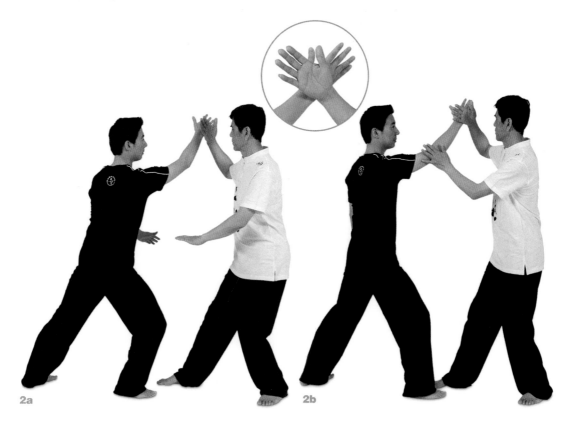

2a 2b

(continued)

3 The white partner continues holding the black partner's elbow tightly with his left hand and makes an internal rotation with his right hand (see figure *a*) to grasp the black partner's right wrist (see figure *b*). The white partner then tries to pull the black partner to the white partner's right side and up so that the black partner may lose his balance. The grasping of the black partner's right hand by the white partner is called *cai* in Chinese.

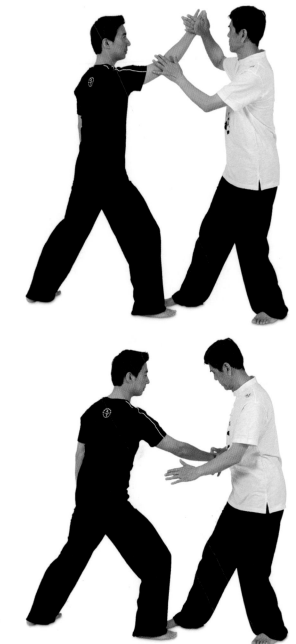

3a

3b

4 To maintain his balance, the black partner naturally pulls his hit back by pulling his right arm down and back, and the white partner releases his grip on the black partner and follows the black partner's pull back to deliver his own hit (see figure *a*). Subsequently, the white partner responds with the same moves that the black partner did in step 2 and pushes forward toward the black partner (see figure *b*). The arm and hand movements of steps 2 through 4 create a vertical circle between the two partners, which is why *vertical circle* is used in the name of this form.

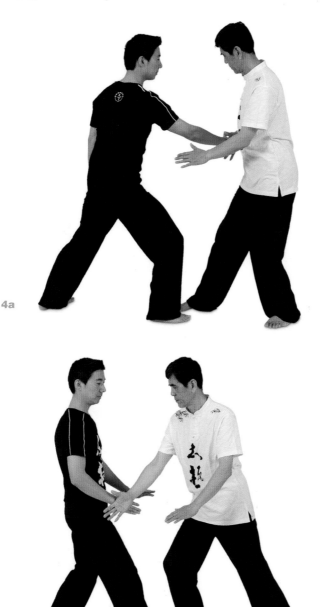

4a

4b

(continued)

5 Repeat steps 2 through 4 until the end of the practice.

6 When finished, both partners move their right legs back to the starting position. Both reach out their arms and then lower them in a relaxed manner to the starting position.

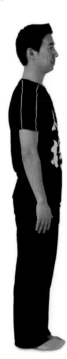

6

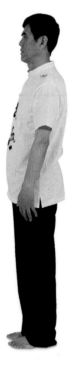

S-Shape *Lu* Push Hands

You learned the *lu* movement, in which you pull both hands back, on page 104 of chapter 7. Now you will learn how to apply that movement with push hands.

1 The white and black partners stand facing each other about 4 to 5 feet (122-152 cm) apart. They separate their legs, the white partner moving his right leg and the black partner moving his left leg. Both take one step forward with their right legs, extending and crossing their right forearms so that the backs of their forearms touch.

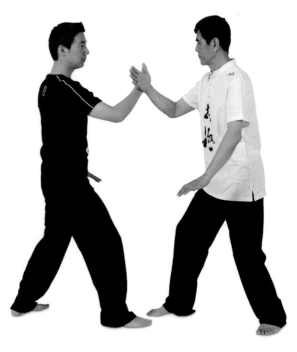

2 The white partner starts to push his right arm forward toward the right side of the black partner's waist by rotating his right arm outward and shifting his body weight onto his front (right) leg at the same time. The black partner tries to deflect the hit by guiding the white partner's hitting right forearm using the back of his right forearm.

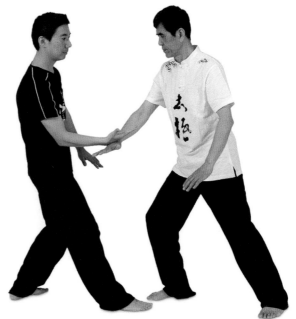

(continued)

3 The black partner grasps with his left hand the white partner's elbow while moving his weight onto his back (left) leg and pulling the white partner's weight to the black partner's right side. To maintain his balance, the white partner pulls his right arm up and back and starts to move his weight onto his back (left) leg. Feeling the white partner pull back, the black partner starts to push up and forward to continue taking advantage of the white partner's momentum.

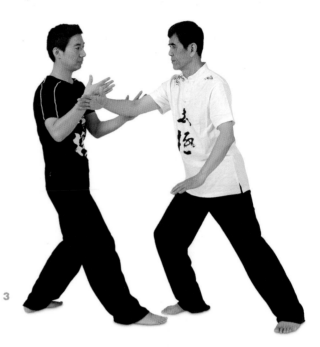

3

4 As in steps 2 and 3, the black partner does an internal rotation of his right arm and pushes forward and down toward the waist of the white partner. To deflect the hit, the white partner guides the black partner's move by using the back of his right arm, grasping the white partner's right elbow with his left hand while moving his weight onto his back (left) leg and pulling the white partner's weight to his right side. This deflection forces the black partner to pull back then to maintain his balance. The movements between partners create an _S_-shaped path that gives this move its name.

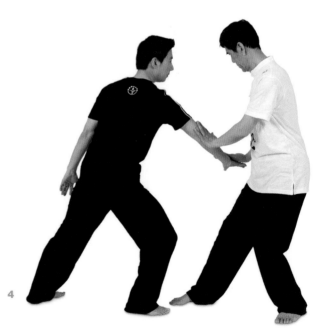

4

5 Steps 2 through 4 can be repeated until the end of the practice.

6 When finished, both partners move their right legs back to the starting position. Both reach out their arms and then lower them in a relaxed manner to the starting position.

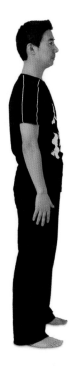

6

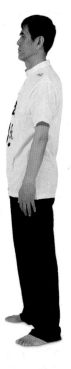

High Cut-Block Push Hands

The name of this push hands form reflects its characteristics. *High* means a push will be performed at or above shoulder level. In tai chi, the movement of hitting your opponent's head using the outer edge of your palm is called *xiao*, which translates to "cut," and using your forearm to block the cut is called *jia*.

1 The white and black partners stand facing each other about 4 to 5 feet (122-152 cm) apart. They start by separating their legs, the white partner moving his right leg and the black partner moving his left leg. Both take one step forward with their right legs, extending and crossing their right forearms so that the backs of their forearms touch.

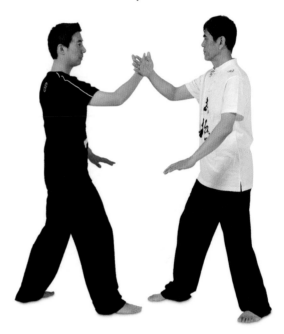

2 The black partner starts to cut the white partner's head with his right hand by moving it forward and up as he shifts his body weight onto the front (right) leg. To protect himself, the white partner tries to block the cut by raising and rotating his right hand (with palm facing himself) and by turning his body to the right while moving his weight onto his back (left) leg.

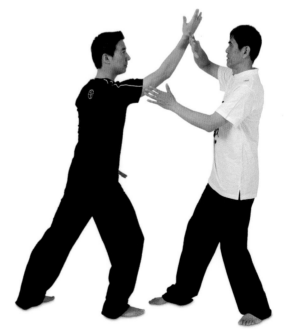

3 Meanwhile, the white partner uses his left hand to grab and press the black partner's elbow, pulling him forward to the white partner's right side so that the black partner might lose his balance.

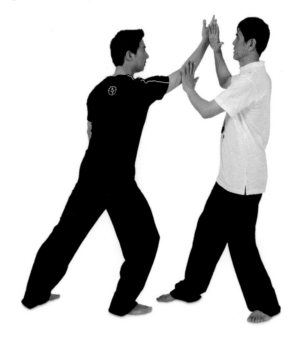

3

(continued)

4 To maintain his balance, the black partner naturally pulls his cut back. The white partner then releases his grasp on the black partner's elbow and follows the black partner's pull back and cut back using his right hand (see figure *a*). In return, the black partner tries to block the white partner's cut by grasping the white partner's elbow with his left hand and pulling the white partner to the black partner's right side (see figure *b*).

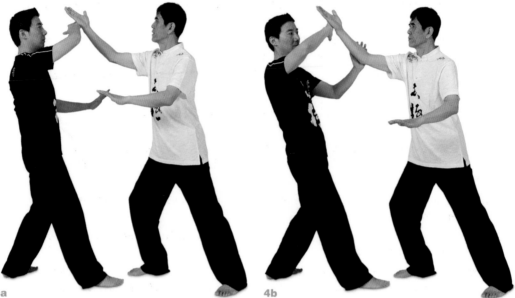

4a   4b

5 Repeat steps 2 through 4 until the end of the practice.

6 When finished, both partners move their right legs back to the starting position. Both reach out their arms and then lower them in a relaxed manner to the starting position.

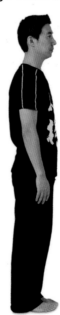

6

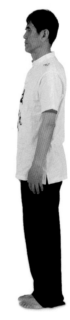

References

American Psychological Association (2012). Stress in America: Our health at risk. Washington, DC: Author.

Centers for Disease Control and Prevention. Falls Among Older Adults. http://www.cdc.gov/HomeandRecreationalSafety/Falls/adultfalls.html

Chen, K.W. (2004) An analytic review of studies measuring effects of external QI in China. *Altern Ther Health Med, 10*(4), 38-50.

Hong, Y. (Ed.). (2008). *Tai chi chuan: State of the art in international research.* New York: Karger.

Martin, Brook I.; Deyo, Richard A.; Mirza, Sohail K; Turner, Judith A.; Comstock, Bryan A.; Hollingworth, William; Sullivan, Sean D. (2008). Expenditures and health status among adults with back and neck problems. *JAMA, 299*(6), 656-664.

Mayo Clinic. Exercise and stress: Get moving to combat stress. http://www.mayoclinic.com/health/exercise-and-stress/SR00036.

Salthous, T.A. (1984). Effects of age and skill in typing. *Journal of Experimental Psychology: General, 113*(3), 345-371.

Schmitz, T. J. (2007). Examination of Sensory Function. In S. B. O'Sullivan & T.J. Schmitz. *Physical Rehabilitation* (5th ed.). Philadelphia, PA: F. A. Davis Company, 121–157.

Stux, G., & Hammerschlag, R. (2001). *Clinical acupuncture: Scientific basis.* New York: Springer.

Wolf, S.L., Barnhart, H.X., Kutner, N.G., McNeely, E., Coogler, C., & Xu, T. (1996). Reducing frailty and falls in older persons: An investigation of t'ai chi and computerized balance training. *Journal of the American Geriatrics Society, 44*(5), 599-600.

Zhu, W., Guan, S., & Yang, Y. (2010). Clinical implication of tai chi interventions: A review. *American Journal of Lifestyle Medicine, 4* (Sept./Oct.), 418-432.

Resources

Publications

Cheng, M. C. (1962). *Tai Chi Chuan: A Method of Calisthenics for Health and Self Defense*. Taipei: Shih Chung Tai-chi Chuan Center.
A translation of a classic text about Tai Chi Chuan by a well-known Chinese tai chi master.

Li, D. (2004). *Taijiquan*. Beijing: Foreign Languages Press: Beijing.
A comprehensive introduction to tai chi by a modern tai chi master.

Websites

www.ncbi.nlm.nih.gov/pubmed/
The database maintained by the US National Library of Medicine at the National Institutes of Health, comprised of more than 21 million citations for biomedical literature, including many current tai chi and health studies.

nccam.nih.gov/health/taichi
The official tai chi information page of the US National Center for Complementary and Alternative Medicine where you can find general information, research spotlights, ongoing medical studies, and scientific literature on tai chi.

www.qigonginstitute.org/html/taichihealth.php
The Qigong Institute website's section on tai chi and health, providing a comprehensive introduction to tai chi and health.

www.worldtaichiday.org/
The official site of World Tai Chi & Qigong Day, where you can find useful information related to tai chi, including events, schools, tips and tutorials, research, and products.

About the Authors

Master Pixiang Qiu is director of the Chinese Wushu (martial arts) Research Center of Shanghai University of Sports. A veteran tai chi instructor, Qiu was named a national master of traditional exercise by the Chinese government. The International Wushu Federation also elected him the first international referee in 1990, named him as one of China's famous wushu professors in 1995, and rated him as a Chinese wushu ninth duan, the highest level in wushu, in 2003. He was the wushu chief judge for the 11th, 12th, 13th, and 14th Asian Games and the chief judge for the 2nd, 4th, and 7th World Wushu Championships. He was designated as an excellent national sports referee and has been ranked as a national top 10 wushu referee.

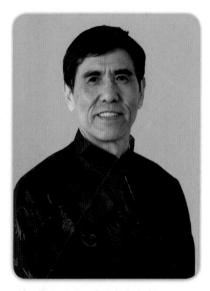

Professor Qiu has published multiple books in Chinese on tai chi and wushu and has lectured worldwide. He gave the keynote address on tai chi at the 2009 American Alliance for Health, Physical Education, Recreation and Dance (AAHPERD) convention and, based on his tai chi teaching and contribution to the promotion of culture exchange, was made an honorary citizen of the city of Dallas in 2009.

Weimo Zhu, PhD, is an internationally known scholar in physical activity and health research at the University of Illinois at Urbana-Champaign, where he regularly teaches mind–body exercise classes at both the university and community levels. He has practiced Chinese mind–body exercises, including tai chi and qigong, for more than 25 years and has been instrumental in introducing them in the United States and around the world. He has given demonstrations and lectures on Chinese mind–body exercises in the United States, China, South Korea, and the Czech Republic. He was awarded a NIH grant to study the effect of long-term mind–body exercise on cancer survivors and presented the research findings at the American College of Sports Medicine (ACSM) annual meetings in 2009.

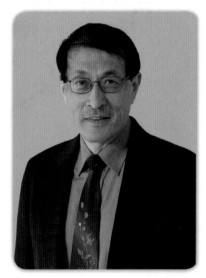

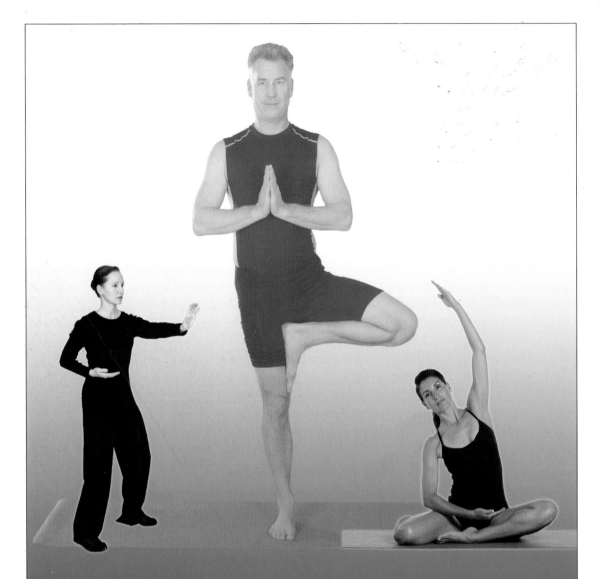
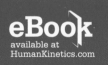